Communication Skills and Challenges in Medical Practice

Editor

HEATHER N. HOFMANN

MEDICAL CLINICS
OF NORTH AMERICA

www.medical.theclinics.com

Consulting Editor
JACK ENDE

July 2022 • Volume 106 • Number 4

ELSEVIER

1600 John F. Kennedy Boulevard • Suite 1800 • Philadelphia, Pennsylvania, 19103-2899

http://www.theclinics.com

MEDICAL CLINICS OF NORTH AMERICA Volume 106, Number 4
July 2022 ISSN 0025-7125, ISBN-13: 978-0-323-98671-7

Editor: Katerina Heidhausen
Developmental Editor: Arlene Campos

Medical Clinics of North America (ISSN 0025-7125) is published bimonthly by Elsevier Inc., 360 Park Avenue South, New York, NY 10010-1710. Months of publication are January, March, May, July, September, and November. Business and editorial offices: 1600 John F. Kennedy Boulevard, Suite 1800, Philadelphia, PA 19103-2899. Periodicals postage paid at New York, NY, and additional mailing offices. Subscription prices are USD $316.00 per year (US individuals), $956.00 per year (US institutions), $100.00 per year (US Students), $396.00 per year (Canadian individuals), $1,004.00 per year (Canadian institutions), $200.00 per year for (foreign students), $100.00 per year for (Canadian students), $439.00 per year (foreign individuals), and $1,004.00 per year (foreign institutions). To receive student/resident rate, orders must be accompanied by name of affiliated institution, date of term, and the signature of program/residency coordinator on institution letterhead. Orders will be billed at individual rate until proof of status is received. Foreign air speed delivery is included in all Clinics' subscription prices. All prices are subject to change without notice. **POSTMASTER:** Send address changes to *Medical Clinics of North America*, Elsevier Health Sciences Division, Subscription Customer Service, 3251 Riverport Lane, Maryland Heights, MO 63043. **Customer Service: Telephone: 1-800-654-2452** (U.S. and Canada); **1-314-447-8871** (outside U.S. and Canada). **Fax: 314-447-8029. E-mail: journalscustomerserviceusa@ elsevier.com** (for print support); **journalsonlinesupport-usa@elsevier.com** (for online support).

Reprints. For copies of 100 or more of articles in this publication, please contact the Commercial Reprints Department, Elsevier Inc., 360 Park Avenue South, New York, NY 10010-1710. Tel.: 212-633-3874; Fax: 212-633-3820; E-mail: reprints@elsevier.com.

Medical Clinics of North America is also published in Spanish by McGraw-Hill Interamericana Editores S. A., P.O. Box 5-237, 06500 Mexico, D.F., Mexico.

Medical Clinics of North America is covered in *MEDLINE/PubMed (Index Medicus), Current Contents, ASCA, Excerpta Medica, Science Citation Index,* and *ISI/BIOMED.*

PROGRAM OBJECTIVE

The goal of the *Medical Clinics of North America* is to keep practicing physicians up to date with current clinical practice by providing timely articles reviewing the state of the art in patient care.

TARGET AUDIENCE

All practicing physicians and other healthcare professionals.

LEARNING OBJECTIVES

Upon completion of this activity, participants will be able to:

1. Review the strategies used to deliver effective provider-patient communication, including the use of technology-enabled communication tools, in promoting patient engagement, patient safety, honest communication, and positive patient outcomes
2. Explain the factors that contribute to the challenges and barriers to effective provider-patient communication.
3. Discuss the advantages of effective provider-patient communication among providers, patients, healthcare systems, and communities.

ACCREDITATION

The Elsevier Office of Continuing Medical Education (EOCME) is accredited by the Accreditation Council for Continuing Medical Education (ACCME) to provide continuing medical education for physicians.

The EOCME designates this journal-based CME activity for a maximum of 15 *AMA PRA Category 1 Credit*(s)™. Physicians should claim only the credit commensurate with the extent of their participation in the activity.

All other healthcare professionals requesting continuing education credit for this enduring material will be issued a certificate of participation.

DISCLOSURE OF CONFLICTS OF INTEREST

The EOCME assesses conflict of interest with its instructors, faculty, planners, and other individuals who are in a position to control the content of CME activities. All relevant conflicts of interest that are identified are thoroughly vetted by EOCME for fair balance, scientific objectivity, and patient care recommendations. EOCME is committed to providing its learners with CME activities that promote improvements or quality in healthcare and not a specific proprietary business or a commercial interest.

The planning committee, staff, authors and editors listed below have identified no financial relationships or relationships to products or devices they or their spouse/life partner have with commercial interest related to the content of this CME activity:
Mazen Al Hammoud; Gopi J. Astik, MD, MS; Moises Auron, MD, FAAP, FACP, SFHM; Maria Barsky, MD; Kasey Boehmer, PhD, MPH, NBC-HWC; David Bustillo; Andrew A. Chang, MD, MPH, MA; Alex Choi, MD; Calvin L. Chou, MD, PhD; Gregorie Constant-Peter, MD, FACP; Sarah Cook, MD; Erin Donovan, PhD; Jessica J. Dreicer, MD; Jessica El Halabi, MD, MBI; Sherrie Flynt Wallington, PhD, MA; Timothy Gilligan, MD; Essa Hariri, MD, MS; David Harris, MD; Heather Hofmann, MD, FACP; Raman Khanna, MD, MAS; Michelle Kittleson, MD, PhD; Anjani Kolahi, MD; Mark A. Lewis, MD; William Minteer, MD; Annecie Noel, DO; Andrew P.J. Olson, MD; Merlin Packiam; Andrew S. Parsons, MD, MPH; R. Ellen Pearlman, MD, FACH; Joseph Rencic, MD; Matthew Sakumoto, MD; Tara Sanft, MD Kevin Shah, MD; Caitlin H. Siropaides, DO; Carl G. Streed, Jr, MD, MPH, FACP; Doreen Thomas-Payne, MSN, BSN, RN, PMHNP-BC; Erin M. Tooley, PhD; Martha Ward, MD; Carli Zegers, PhD, MBA, APRN, FNP-BC

UNAPPROVED/OFF-LABEL USE DISCLOSURE

The EOCME requires CME faculty to disclose to the participants;

1. When products or procedures being discussed are off-label, unlabelled, experimental, and/or investigational (not US Food and Drug Administration [FDA] approved); and
2. Any limitations on the information presented, such as data that are preliminary or that represent ongoing research, interim analyses, and/or unsupported opinions. Faculty may discuss information about pharmaceutical agents that is outside of FDA-approved labelling. This information is intended solely for CME and is not intended to promote off-label use of these medications. If you have any questions, contact the medical affairs department of the manufacturer for the most recent prescribing information.

TO ENROLL

To enroll in the *Medical Clinics of North America* Continuing Medical Education program, call customer service at 1-800-654-2452 or sign up online at http://www.theclinics.com/home/cme. The CME program is available to subscribers for an additional annual fee of USD 324.00.

METHOD OF PARTICIPATION

In order to claim credit, participants must complete the following;

1. Complete enrolment as indicated above.
2. Read the activity.
3. Complete the CME Test and Evaluation. Participants must achieve a score of 70% on the test. All CME Tests and Evaluations must be completed online.

CME INQUIRIES/SPECIAL NEEDS

For all CME inquiries or special needs, please contact elsevierCME@elsevier.com.

MEDICAL CLINICS OF NORTH AMERICA

FORTHCOMING ISSUES

September 2022
Nutrition in the Practice of Medicine:
A Practical Approach
David S. Seres, *Editor*

November 2022
Clinical Psychiatry
Leo Sher, *Editor*

January 2023
Pulmonary Diseases
Daniel M. Goodenberger, *Editor*

RECENT ISSUES

May 2022
Disease-Based Physical Examination
Paul Aronowitz, *Editor*

March 2022
Update in Preventive Cardiology
Douglas S. Jacoby, *Editor*

January 2022
Substance Use Disorders
Melissa B. Weimer, *Editor*

Contributors

CONSULTING EDITOR

JACK ENDE, MD, MACP
The Schaeffer Professor of Medicine, Perelman School of Medicine, University of Pennsylvania, Philadelphia, Pennsylvania, USA

EDITOR

HEATHER N. HOFMANN, MD, FACP
Associate Staff Physician, Department of Hospital Medicine, Cleveland Clinic Foundation, Assistant Professor, Cleveland Clinic Lerner College of Medicine at Case Western Reserve University, Cleveland, Ohio, USA

AUTHORS

MAZEN AL HAMMOUD, BS
Gilbert and Rose-Marie Chagoury School of Medicine, Lebanese American University, Byblos, Lebanon

GOPI J. ASTIK, MD, MS
Assistant Professor of Medicine, Division of Hospital Medicine, Northwestern University Feinberg School of Medicine, Chicago, Illinois, USA

MOISES AURON, MD, FAAP, FACP, SFHM
Staff, Departments of Hospital Medicine and Pediatric Hospital Medicine, Professor of Medicine and Pediatrics, Cleveland Clinic Lerner College of Medicine at Case Western Reserve University, Cleveland Clinic, Cleveland, Ohio, USA

MARIA BARSKY, MD
Assistant Professor, Hospitalist Program, UC Irvine Medical Center, Orange, California, USA

KASEY R. BOEHMER, PhD, MPH, NBC-HWC
Division of Health Care Delivery Research, Knowledge and Evaluation Research (KER) Unit, Mayo Clinic, Rochester, Minnesota, USA

DAVID BUSTILLO, MS4
University of California, Irvine School of Medicine, Irvine, California, USA

ANDREW A. CHANG, MD, MPH, MA
Clinical Assistant Professor, Department of Medicine, State University of New York Downstate, NYC Health + Hospitals/Kings County, Brooklyn, New York, USA

ALEX CHOI, MD
Instructor of Medicine, Yale Palliative Care Program, Yale New Haven Hospital, New Haven, Connecticut, USA

CALVIN L. CHOU, MD, PhD
Professor of Clinical Medicine, University of California and Veterans Affairs Healthcare System, San Francisco, California, USA

GREGORIE CONSTANT-PETER, MD, FAAFP
Orange County Government, Florida, Corrections Health Services, Orlando, Florida, USA

SARAH COOK, MD
Assistant Professor, Department of Psychiatry and Behavioral Sciences, Emory University School of Medicine, Atlanta, Georgia, USA

ERIN DONOVAN, PhD
Department of Communication Studies, The University of Texas at Austin, Austin, Texas, USA

JESSICA J. DREICER, MD
Department of Medicine, University of Virginia, Charlottesville, Virginia, USA

JESSICA EL HALABI, MD, MBI
Internal Medicine Department, Cleveland Clinic, Cleveland, Ohio, USA

TIMOTHY GILLIGAN, MD
Department of Hematology and Medical Oncology, Cleveland Clinic Taussig Cancer Institute, Cleveland, Ohio, USA

ESSA HARIRI, MD, MS
Department of Internal Medicine, Cleveland Clinic Foundation, Cleveland, Ohio, USA

DAVID HARRIS, MD
Department of Palliative and Supportive Care, Cleveland Clinic Taussig Cancer Institute, Cleveland, Ohio, USA

HEATHER N. HOFMANN, MD, FACP
Associate Staff Physician, Department of Hospital Medicine, Cleveland Clinic Foundation, Assistant Professor, Cleveland Clinic Lerner College of Medicine at Case Western Reserve University, Cleveland, Ohio, USA

RAMAN KHANNA, MD, MAS
Associate Professor of Clinical Medicine, Department of Medicine, University of California, San Francisco, San Francisco, California, USA

MICHELLE M. KITTLESON, MD, PhD
Department of Cardiology, Smidt Heart Institute, Cedars-Sinai Medical Center, Los Angeles, California, USA

ANJANI KOLAHI, MD
University of California, Irvine Medical Center, Orange, California, USA

MARK A. LEWIS, MD
Intermountain Healthcare, Murray, Utah, USA

WILLIAM MINTEER, MD
Division of Community Internal Medicine, Mayo Clinic, Rochester, Minnesota, USA

ANNECIE NOEL, DO
Chief Resident, Department of Medicine, Memorial Sloan Kettering Cancer Center, New York, New York, USA

ANDREW P.J. OLSON, MD, FACP, FAAP
Associate Professor of Medicine, Section of Hospital Medicine, Division of General Internal Medicine, Department of Medicine, Division of Pediatric Hospital Medicine, Department of Pediatrics, University of Minnesota Medical School, Minneapolis, Minnesota, USA

ANDREW S. PARSONS, MD, MPH
Department of Medicine, University of Virginia, Charlottesville, Virginia, USA

RUTH ELLEN BLEDSOE PEARLMAN, MD, FACH
Donald and Barbara Zucker School of Medicine at Hofstra/Northwell, Hempstead, New York, USA

JOSEPH RENCIC, MD
Department of Medicine, Boston University, Boston, Massachusetts, USA

MATTHEW SAKUMOTO, MD
Adjunct Clinical Professor, Department of Medicine, University of California, San Francisco, San Francisco, California, USA

TARA SANFT, MD
Associate Professor of Medicine (Medical Oncology), Chief, Patient Experience Officer, Medical Director, Survivorship Clinic, Yale New Haven Hospital, New Haven, Connecticut, USA

KEVIN SHAH, MD
Department of Medicine, Division of Cardiology, University of Utah Hospital, Salt Lake City, Utah, USA

CAITLIN H. SIROPAIDES, DO
Assistant Professor, Department of Internal Medicine, Section of Supportive and Palliative Care, The University of Texas Southwestern Medical Center, Dallas, Texas, USA

CARL G. STREED Jr, MD, MPH, FACP
Assistant Professor of Medicine, Section of General Internal Medicine, Department of Medicine, Boston University School of Medicine, Research Lead, Center for Transgender Medicine and Surgery, Boston Medical Center, Boston, Massachusetts, USA

ERIN M. TOOLEY, PhD
Department of Psychology and Public Health, Roger Williams University, Bristol, Rhode Island, USA

SHERRIE FLYNT WALLINGTON, PhD, MA
Assistant Professor of Health Disparities and Oncology, George Washington University, School of Nursing, Washington, DC, USA

MARTHA WARD, MD
Associate Professor, Departments of Psychiatry and Behavioral Sciences, and Medicine, Emory University School of Medicine, Atlanta, Georgia, USA

CARLI ZEGERS, PhD, MBA, APRN, FNP-BC
Assistant Professor of Nursing, University of Kansas, Kansas City, Kansas, USA

Contents

Foreword: Improving Our Communication Skills: More Than We Know   xv

Jack Ende

Preface: Tomato Tomahto   xvii

Heather N. Hofmann

Essential Elements of Communication   557

Heather N. Hofmann, Gregorie Constant-Peter, and Ruth Ellen Bledsoe Pearlman

> Relationship-centered communication (RCC) is an effective approach to patient-provider communication. This article describes RCC components known as the essential elements of communication. The article also describes current standard conceptual models for applying RCC to the patient encounter, including a structure for relationship building. The authors also explore the challenges to using RCC.

Patient Perspective: Importance and How to Elicit   569

Mark A. Lewis and David Bustillo

> The authors present models for patient care, reflecting on its modernization. A review of technology including electronic health records is provided, noting its benefits and constraints on the patient-clinician relationship. Keeping in mind the fact that patients are the "end users" of health care systems, several approaches to improving patient experience are shared.

Addressing the Challenges of Cross-Cultural Communication   577

Carli Zegers and Moises Auron

> Cross-cultural communication has many challenges due to the complexity of culture, communication, and language. Improving cross-cultural communication in health care is critical to reducing disparities and improving health equity. Specifically, improving cross-cultural communication must be prioritized to overcome systemic barriers and to eliminate disparities that stem from stigma and biases. Communication must be improved, ideally via a cultural humility framework. Unconscious bias and communication training must be intentional. Culture is an attribute and should be celebrated and incorporated into health practice at all levels to prioritize health equity.

Health Communication and Sexual Orientation, Gender Identity, and Expression   589

Carl G. Streed Jr.

> The purpose of this article is to provide guidance on completing a thorough, competent, and culturally appropriate health history with details

specific to the care of lesbian, gay, bisexual, transgender, queer, intersex, and asexual (LGBTQIA) persons and communities.

The Diagnostic Medical Interview   601

Jessica J. Dreicer, Andrew S. Parsons, and Joseph Rencic

The diagnostic medical interview spans from the chief concern to the formation of a differential diagnosis. The patient's unique expression of their symptoms is the central component of this conversation. The interview should begin by eliciting the patient's chief concern with an open-ended question and then move through three nonlinear phases: open-ended elicitation, guided elicitation, and hypothesis-driven elicitation. Performing a comprehensive medical interview by obtaining background health information and the review of systems can help to expand or shrink the differential diagnosis. Clinicians should elicit information about specific symptoms and background information with a significant likelihood to narrow the differential diagnosis.

Identifying and Managing Treatment Nonadherence   615

Jessica El Halabi, William Minteer, and Kasey R. Boehmer

Nonadherence to medical treatment is exceptionally common and associated with poor clinical outcomes, a negative impact on quality of life, and a large financial burden on health care systems. This article first addresses key contributors to nonadherence from patient-specific, treatment-specific, and health care system–specific factors. Second, it outlines tools for the practicing clinician to identify, evaluate, and manage nonadherence across the spectrum of chronic disease in partnership with patients.

Motivating Behavioral Change   627

Erin M. Tooley and Anjani Kolahi

Motivational interviewing (MI) allows medical providers and patients to have more productive conversations about changing health behaviors. MI helps patients talk themselves into changing by evoking discussion around change, thus resolving natural ambivalence. MI practitioners cultivate a spirit of MI and use specific skills and strategies to develop discrepancy between the patient's current behavior and their goals or values. This article discusses the flow of MI, the spirit and method of MI including specific skills and strategies, and important considerations in implementing MI.

Delivering Bad News   641

David Harris and Timothy Gilligan

Giving bad news is a recurrent and predictable task in our lives as humans interacting with other humans. This article presents frameworks and best practices that can help us to deliver bad news in health care in a way that is experienced as caring and empathic, and supports the patient as they adjust to their new reality. Key skills include responding to patients' emotions empathically, leading with an exploration of the patient's understanding and expectations, delivering the bad news clearly and concisely, and individualizing the balance of empathy and support with providing information and developing a plan.

Establishing Goals of Care

653

Alex Choi and Tara Sanft

Establishing goals of care (GOC) is a crucial component of a patient's treatment plan. The need for better physician-patient communication in this area has been recognized for decades, yet several gaps remain. Challenges exist for both physician and patient. Physicians should pursue a patient-led approach, exercise cultural competency, and use various communication techniques to guide patients when establishing GOC.

The Role of Informed Consent in Clinical and Research Settings

663

Essa Hariri, Mazen Al Hammoud, Erin Donovan, Kevin Shah, and Michelle M. Kittleson

Informed consent plays an integral role in governing the patient-physician relationship with origins traced back to ancient Greek philosophy. The main pillars of informed consent are autonomy, integrity, respect, and care. In the last century, these notions have been codified into legislation to promote healthy patient-physician relationships. Understanding the process of informed consent is critical for patients, researchers, and medical practitioners. In this article, the authors provide a brief historical narrative of informed consent, elaborate on the process of obtaining an ethically and legally valid informed consent, and present some of the future challenges in the field.

Classifying and Disclosing Medical Errors

675

Maria Barsky, Andrew P.J. Olson, and Gopi J. Astik

Medical errors are an unfortunate but common occurrence in health care. It is important to understand what medical errors are and what types of harm can occur to patients. Along with recognition of the error, disclosure is an equally important part of the process. Clinicians should provide open and honest discussion about the events that occurred to patients along with feedback to institutions on ways to prevent such errors in the future.

When Communication Breaks Down: Handling Hostile Patients

689

Martha Ward and Sarah Cook

Difficult patient encounters are common in clinical practice, with many arising from patient hostility owing to a breakdown in communication and the health care alliance. Patient anger may be a manifestation of fear, grief, or discontent with prior experiences in the health care system, but there may also be contributions from specific patient, physician, or situational factors. Physicians may intervene with specific actions based on these individual factors, while focusing on self-reflection to better understand their part in creating a hostile physician-patient dyad.

Using Technology to Enhance Communication   705

Matthew Sakumoto and Raman Khanna

> Digital communication, facilitated by the rise of the electronic health record and telehealth, has transformed clinical workflow. The communication tools, and the purposes they are being used for, need to account for the benefits, risks, and fault tolerance for each tool. In this article, the authors offer several suggestions on how to approach these important issues. These new digital communication tools open the door to novel care models for connecting patients and providers. Most importantly, the way a message is delivered, not the medium through which it is transmitted, is the key to successful communication.

Communicating with Community: Health Disparities and Health Equity Considerations   715

Sherrie Flynt Wallington and Annecie Noel

> This article explores why communicating with communities is important to the health of individuals as well as public health, and best practices of how. We outline the use of relevant theoretic frameworks, understanding the role of technological contextual changes, trust despite misinformation, health and digital literacy skills, and working with the community for effective reciprocal communication. Strategies for developing community communication are also enumerated and applied to addressing health disparities.

Improving Communication Skills: A Roadmap for Humanistic Health Care   727

Andrew A. Chang, Caitlin H. Siropaides, and Calvin L. Chou

> This article outlines frameworks that enable health care providers to take steps to improve their health care communication skills, including not only outward-facing conversational tools but also personal awareness. Such awareness includes recognition of bias and emotional reactions, their behavioral consequences, and how to intervene when necessary. The authors describe the intrinsic and extrinsic motivators to improving communication skills, followed by a review of foundational communication microskills and suggestions on how to improve them through the perspectives of the clinician as a self-learner, the clinician with external coaching, and the administrator/leader.

Foreword

Improving Our Communication Skills: More Than We Know

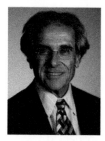

Jack Ende, MD, MACP
Consulting Editor

Physician-patient communication, framed as a set of skills that lie at the core of medical practice, is different from other skill sets that clinicians must master. Why? Because we assume we already know how to communicate. What is there to learn?

We humbly enter, as medical students, our physical diagnosis course, or, as experienced practitioners, our point-of-care ultrasound course. We freely admit we are novices at detecting a third heart sound or identifying a pleural infusion. Nothing to be ashamed of here, and nothing to unlearn.

Communication is different. We communicated before we became doctors and nurses, and we continue to communicate when our office hours end. What more, we may ask, do we need to learn about communication in medical practice? I say, *more than we know*.

I came to this realization, and am so enthusiastic about this particular issue of *Medical Clinics of North America*, because I have made almost all the mistakes. I have missed gaining insight into my patients' perspectives; failed to appreciate nonadherence, or addressed it skillfully when I have appreciated it; done a less-than-stellar job motivating behavioral change; stammered my way through delivering bad news, or avoided that discussion entirely; done a poor job of handling the angry or hostile patient; and procrastinated in establishing goals of care. In short, I have exemplified, hopefully more in the past than in the present, the rationale for taking seriously the specific and instrumental skills that are addressed by Guest Editor, Heather Hoffman, and her expert authors. Over the course of my career, I have come to appreciate that communication skills in medical practice depend upon, first, acknowledging that there's a great deal to learn; second, that we are not as expert as we think we are; and finally, that communication skills pave the way for more effective patient outcomes.

Med Clin N Am 106 (2022) xv–xvi
https://doi.org/10.1016/j.mcna.2022.04.001
0025-7125/22/© 2022 Published by Elsevier Inc.

So, dig in. Use this issue as a checklist to help you identify areas of strength and weakness, and try out the tools and techniques that the experts recommend. I believe this will be time well spent.

Jack Ende, MD, MACP
The Schaeffer Professor of Medicine
Perelman School of Medicine of the
University of Pennsylvania
5033 West Gates Pavilion
3400 Spruce Street
Philadelphia, PA 19104, USA

E-mail address:
jack.ende@pennmedicine.upenn.edu

Preface

Tomato Tomahto

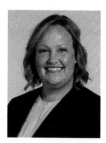

Heather N. Hofmann, MD, FACP
Editor

Modern medicine is complicated. In the early 1800s, doctors placed a shingle above their office entrance. In a single examination room, the physician would sit, communicate, and heal. In the twenty-first century, those shingles are bright hospital lights, Web site banners, building directories near the elevator, and perhaps, still, shingles. Eventually, the patient finds us, or we find them. We sit. We communicate. We heal. Which parts of traditional healthcare communication are timeless? Which parts are new? This unique issue of *Medical Clinics of North America* shares evidence-based approaches to healthcare communication. Allow these authors to help make modern patient interactions better for the patient and care team.

Unprecedented. COVID-19 is a novel disease. In many ways the COVID-19 pandemic is unprecedented for the global population and modern medical field. Most front-line clinicians have had the unprecedented task of performing the diagnostic interview, delivering bad news, and establishing goals of care while speaking through personal protective equipment and with patients' loved ones remotely via video conference. To a previously healthy patient, a new cancer diagnosis is unprecedented. The scans, the procedures, the infusions—uncharted territory, wrought with uncertainty. Precedent tells us that novelty and challenges in medicine are commonplace.

High value. High-value care benefits the patient and minimizes financial cost and harm. With innovative diagnostics and therapies, as well as the globalization of healthcare, patients want the best care, and we want what is best for them and the system. Sometimes we are on the same page and sometimes we are not. As part of informed consent, providers must assess if the chosen care plan aligns with a patient's value system. What are the patient's values?

Personalized medicine. Genetics has a role in guiding the prevention, diagnosis, and treatment of some diseases. Science is at the core of personalized medicine. In healthcare communication, the phrase "personalized medicine" parallels "person-centered language." In the words of Norman Cousins, "It is the physician's respect for the human soul that determines the worth of his science."[1] Are we speaking effectively to patients of other cultures or gender identity? How do we talk to patients when we've made a mistake? Science is not perfect, and science is fluid. We as clinicians can improve our communication skills.

Provider. Approximately one in five inpatients can name the physician in charge of their care; most inpatients cannot. Provider teams include licensed physicians, trainees, students, and advanced practice providers. Are we going to refer to ourselves as doctors? Clinicians? Physicians? Providers? How can we help patients if they don't even know who we are?

This unique issue brings together a breadth of experts in healthcare communication, a field that expands beyond physicians. The authors insight into the practice of modern medicine is of paramount significance. They have volunteered their time at a time when time is sacred. I appreciate their dedication and contributions.

Thank you also to my family for their support as this project ripened. You enrich my growth as a physician, even if tomatoes are no longer your favorite.

While our profession is challenged, communication is our stronghold. I hope this information resonates with your medical practice and teaches you something new. We are lifelong learners, after all.

Heather N. Hofmann, MD, FACP
Associate Staff Physician
Department of Hospital Medicine
Cleveland Clinic Foundation; Assistant Professor
Cleveland Clinic Lerner College of Medicine at Case Western Reserve University
9500 Euclid Avenue, M75
Cleveland, OH 44118, USA

E-mail address:
heather.n.hofmann@gmail.com

REFERENCES

1. Cousins N. The physician as communicator. JAMA 1982;248(5):587–9.

Essential Elements of Communication

Heather Hofmann, MD, FACP[a], Gregorie Constant-Peter, MD, FAAFP[b], Ruth Ellen Bledsoe Pearlman, MD, FACH[c,1,*]

KEYWORDS

- Communication • Physician-patient relations • Relationship-centered
- Patient-centered care • Health care • Health communication

KEY POINTS

- Relationship-centered care recognizes that all health care relationships occur in the context of reciprocal influence, include the dimensions of personhood in addition to roles, and involve affect and emotion.
- Relationship-centered care improves outcomes for patients, providers, and institutions.
- Communication skills are essential to relationship-centered and patient-centered care.
- Experts in health care communication reached consensus about which skills are considered essential, and several models incorporate these skills.
- Essential communication skills include active listening without interruption, the use of open-ended questions to explore the patients' concerns and assess understanding, the use of plain language and summary, and the ability to respond to emotion with expressed empathy.

INTRODUCTION

"Questions, connections and common ground are vital tools in assisting your patient to feel like a whole person, and helping them remember you are too."
                              -Marcus Engel, The Other End of the Stethoscope

The concept of relationship-centered care stems from the patient-centered care movement of recent decades.[1] Patient-centered care prioritizes patient preferences, improves quality of care, and supports morally, ethically sound medical practice.[2] The Pew-Fetzer Task Force helped to define relationship-centered care as patient-centered, with a focus on the meaningful relationship between patient and clinician.[3] **Box 1** lists the core principles of relationship-centered care.[4]

---

[a] Cleveland Clinic Foundation, 9500 Euclid Avenue, M75, Cleveland, OH 44195, USA; [b] Orange County Government, Florida, Corrections Health Services, 3855 S John Young Parkway, Orlando, FL 32839, USA; [c] Donald and Barbara Zucker School of Medicine at Hofstra/Northwell, 500 Hofstra Boulevard, Hempstead, NY 11549, USA
[1] Contributing author.
* Corresponding author.
E-mail address: r.e.pearlman@hofstra.edu

Med Clin N Am 106 (2022) 557–567
https://doi.org/10.1016/j.mcna.2022.01.004
0025-7125/22/© 2022 Elsevier Inc. All rights reserved.

medical.theclinics.com

Box 1
Principles of relationship-centered care

1. Relationships in health care ought to include dimensions of personhood as well as roles
2. Affect and emotion are important components of relationships in health care
3. All health care relationships occur in the context of reciprocal influence
4. Relationship-centered care has a moral foundation

To excel at relationship-centered care, one must build and hone knowledge, skills, and attitudes in 4 areas (**Box 2**).[3] These 4 areas are interdependent. Relationship-centered communication (RCC) is an approach that a provider can use to incorporate the principles of relationship-centered care in their communication with patients.

RCC has positive effects on patients, providers, and the health care system. Patient-centered communication techniques can reduce pain and anxiety, promote weight loss, and reduce systolic blood pressure.[5–11] For hospital-based physicians, RCC elicits clinically relevant information and contributes to patient agreement about treatment plans.[12] RCC increases communication ratings for physicians and does not prolong the encounter.[13] Studies have shown that physicians are happier when RCC is used. Both patient and provider benefits impact the health care system as a whole.

CURRENT EVIDENCE
Essential Elements

How does a provider practice or perform RCC? As with any skill or procedure, understanding the components of RCC is crucial. These components are known as the essential elements of physician-patient communication. In 1999, a group of people from medical schools, residency programs, continuing medical education providers, and prominent medical educational organizations in North America met to identify and specifically articulate ways to facilitate communication teaching, assessment, and evaluation.[14] The group created the Kalamazoo Consensus Statement.[14] The Kalamazoo Consensus Statement delineates a set of essential elements in physician-patient communication. These elements were intended to facilitate the development, implementation, and evaluation of communication-oriented curricula in medical education and inform the development of specific standards in this domain.

The essential elements are best delineated as communication tasks (**Table 1**). The task of building a relationship is fundamental and occurs within and across encounters. The other communication tasks are more sequential. These essential elements can be applied to multiple care settings and patient encounters.

Box 2
Knowledge, skills, and attitudes that pertain to the patient-provider relationship

1. Self-awareness and continuing self-growth
2. Patient's experience of health and illness
3. Developing and maintaining relationships with patients
4. Communicating clearly and effectively

Table 1
Essential elements of communication

Communication Task	Examples of Relevant Knowledge, Skills, and Attitudes
Build a relationship	Greet and show interest in patient as a person
	Use words that show care and concern throughout interview
	Use tone, pace, eye contact, and posture that show care and concern
Open the discussion	Allow patient to complete opening statement without interruption
	Elicit patient's full set of concerns
	Explain and/or negotiate an agenda for visit
Gather information	Use open-ended and closed-ended questions appropriately
	Structure, clarify, and summarize information
	Actively listen using nonverbal (eg, eye contact) and verbal (eg, words of encouragement) techniques
Understand the patient's perspective	Explore contextual factors (eg, family, culture, gender, age, socioeconomic status, spirituality)
	Explore beliefs, concerns, and expectations about health and illness
	Acknowledge and respond to patient's ideas, feelings, and values
Share information	Use language patient can understand
	Check for understanding
	Encourage questions
Reach agreement on problems and plans	Encourage patient to participate in decisions to the extent he or she desires
	Check patient's willingness and ability to follow plan
	Identify and enlist resources and support
Provide closure	Ask whether patient has other issues or concerns
	Summarize and affirm agreement with plan of action
	Discuss follow-up (eg, next visit, plan for unexpected outcomes)

Adapted from Kalamazoo Consensus Statement[14] and Essential Elements Communication Checklist.[25]

An example of the opening and closing of an encounter using relationship-centered skills in the outpatient setting is given. The following dialogue is annotated to demonstrate the essential elements of communication.

Example: The opening of a new patient encounter with a primary care provider.

Provider: "Hi. Mrs. Smith? I am Dr. Jones-it is great to meet you. Just to make sure I have the right chart; can you confirm your name and date of birth?" [Build a Relationship: Greet]

Patient: "Yes. Margaret Smith, 12/10/1963."

Provider: "Terrific, I have the right chart. I am just going to wash my hands before we start." (as washing hands) "I noticed your shirt says "Grandma knows best." How many grandkids do you have?" [Build a Relationship: Show interest in patient as a person]

Patient: "My daughter has 2 boys, and my son has a new baby girl born a month ago!"

Provider: "Congratulations! People say being a grandparent is even more amazing than being a parent." [Build a Relationship: Use words that show care and concern throughout interview] Patient: "That's for sure. And I am lucky they all live nearby so I get to see them a lot."

Provider: "That is lucky! Is it ok if I take a seat?" [Build a Relationship: Use words that show care and concern throughout interview]

Patient: "Of course."

Provider: "First, I just want to acknowledge the computer—I will need to do some typing for my records, but I will do my best to keep it to a minimum so that I can focus my attention on you." [Build a Relationship: Use eye contact that shows care and concern]

Patient: "Great."

Provider: "How can I help you today?" [Gather information: Use open-ended questions]

Patient: "I have been having a lot of back pain recently. I've had it on and off for a couple of years, but it seems like it has been increasing in intensity lately and happening more frequently." [Open the Discussion: Allow the patient to complete opening statement without interruption]

Provider: "I am sorry to hear that. Before we jump into the story of the back pain I just want to make sure I get a list of all the concerns you were hoping to cover today. What else is on your mind?" [Open the Discussion: Elicit full set of concerns]

Patient: "Well. I do need a refill of my blood pressure meds."

Provider: "Sure thing. So back pain, blood pressure meds...what else?" [Open the Discussion: Elicit full set of concerns]

Patient: "I have been feeling a little down lately and having trouble sleeping."

Provider: "Thank you for sharing that. You do seem a little down, and it can be so hard to have trouble sleeping. We will definitely spend some time on that. What else is on your mind?" [Build a Relationship: Use words that show care and concern throughout the interview; Open the Discussion: Elicit full set of concerns]

Patient: "That's enough!"

Provider: "Alright. So, we have back pain, blood pressure meds, feeling down, and trouble sleeping. I would also like to review what vaccinations and screening tests you are due for if that is alright?" [Open the Discussion: Explain and/or negotiate an agenda for the visit]

Patient: "Of course."

Provider: "Of the three concerns you mentioned, which is most important to you today?" [Build a Relationship: Negotiate an agenda]

Patient: "Well actually I think feeling down and having trouble sleeping really started with the back pain so maybe we should start there?"

Provider: "Sounds good. Why don't you tell me the story of the back pain, starting with when it first began and taking me through to now?" [Gather Information: Use open-ended questions]

Patient: "Well, like I said, I have had pain in my lower back for the last couple of years, usually related to overdoing my workout without stretching enough or when I am unusually stressed. I take a couple of Advil and do more stretching, maybe take a day off of exercising and it goes away. For the past couple of weeks, though, it has gotten worse. It started when I was trying to help my daughter move- I was lifting some heavy boxes and felt my lower back spasm. I went home, took some Advil, put a heating pad on it, but it didn't go away. Since then, I have noticed that the pain now shoots down my left buttock. It is pretty much there all the time now." [Open the Discussion: Allow the patient to complete opening statement without interruption]

Provider: "That sounds really difficult." [Build a Relationship: Use words that show care and concern throughout the interview] "How has this impacted your life?" [Understand the Patient's Perspective: Explore contextual factors]

Patient: "Well, I can't exercise at all. It makes it hard to fall asleep and stay asleep at night so I am exhausted during the day."

Provider: "That sounds really debilitating." [Build a Relationship: Use words that show care and concern throughout the interview] "What do you think might be causing the pain? [Understand the Patient's Perspective: Explore beliefs, concerns, and expectations about health and illness]

Patient: "My husband has a slipped disc in his lower back and has had the same kind of pain in the past, so I am worried I might have that too."

Provider: "Yes, it certainly has a similar pattern. What concerns you the most?"

Patient: "I am worried it won't go away, and that I'll have to get surgery."

Provider: "I think most people in your situation would be concerned about that. I am so glad that you came in today. We will definitely get to the bottom of this and get you feeling better as soon as possible, and hopefully without needing surgery!" [Understand the Patient's Perspective: Acknowledge and respond to the patient's ideas, feelings, and values]

Patient: "Thank you, that would be amazing."

Provider: "Let me just make sure I've got the story right; please correct me if I am wrong. You have had pain in the lower back on and off for years, usually from overdoing it with exercise, sometimes from stress, but it is usually relieved with Advil or stretching or resting. This pain is a little different in that it started when you were lifting boxes helping your daughter move. You had an immediate back spasm followed by a constant pain that now shoots down the back of your left leg and doesn't go away with Advil, stretching, rest, or heat. It prevents you from exercising and makes it hard to get enough sleep, so you are pretty exhausted. Did I get that right?" [Gather information: Structure, clarify, and summarize information]

Patient: "Yes!"

Provider: "And all of this has led you to feel pretty down, is that right? Shall we talk a little more about that?"

Fast forward to the closing of the visit, after gathering the full history and completing the physical examination: Provider: "So your examination is consistent with what we would call a "herniated disc." I know you said that your husband had a "slipped disc" in the past. What do you understand about a "slipped" or "herniated disc?" [Share information: Check for understanding]

Patient: "I know it has something to do with the nerves from the spine in the lower back."

Provider: "That's exactly right. To understand what a herniated disc is and how it causes symptoms, it's helpful to first learn a little about the back and spine. The back is made up of vertebrae that sit on top of one another like a stack of coins. Each bone has a hole in the center. When stacked, the holes in the bones form a hollow "tube" that protects the spinal cord. The spinal cord is like a highway of nerves that connects the brain to the rest of the body. The spinal cord runs through the tube and nerves branch out from the spinal cord and pass in between each vertebrae to connect to parts of the body. Cartilage discs sit in between each of the vertebrae to add cushioning. Sometimes these discs slip out of position and press on the nerves, causing pain. Sometimes the outer shell of the discs breaks open, spilling the jelly material inside which irritates nearby nerves." [Share information: Use language the patient can understand] "What questions do you have about that?" [Share information: Encourage questions]

Patient: "So did the heavy lifting cause the disc to slip?"

Provider: "Possibly, though many times it can just happen out of the blue."

Patient: "So what is the next step?"

Provider: "The good news is that you don't have any of the warning signs of something more serious going on, so we don't need to do any imaging unless the pain doesn't go away. I also think you have been under-using the ibuprofen, so we have room to go up on the amount and frequency of that. Sometimes patients also benefit from either physical therapy or acupuncture or chiropractic adjustment. What are your thoughts on those options?" [Reach Agreement on Problems and Plans: Encourage the patient to participate in decisions to the extent he or she desires]

Patient: "I would be willing to try some physical therapy. I don't like the thought of acupuncture and my husband didn't have a great experience with a chiropractor."

Provider: "Alright. So, let's try increasing the ibuprofen to 600 mg four times a day with food to protect your stomach. I will also write you a prescription for physical therapy. I would like to see you back in two weeks to check in on the pain control, but obviously I would want to hear back from you sooner if things get worse." [Provide Closure: Discuss follow-up] "What questions do you have?" [Share information: Encourage questions]

Patient: "Should I continue to avoid exercising?"

Provider: "Yes. I would hold off on exercise for now but am confident we will be able to get you back to your normal routine soon. What other questions do you have?" [Share information: Encourage questions]

Patient: "No more questions for now. I feel relieved to have a plan."

Provider: "Me too! I know we have covered a lot of information in the last few minutes. Just so I know that I have been clear, would you mind reviewing what you understand about the problem and the plan going forward?" [Share information: Check for understanding]

Patient: "Well, my pain is being caused by a slipped disc, which is when one of the discs that cushions the back bones of the spine slips and compresses the nerves or when one of them breaks open and the inside spills out and irritates the nerve. It may or may not have been caused by the heavy lifting I was doing helping my daughter move."

Provider: "Perfect! And what's the plan?"

Patient: "I don't need any imaging because I don't have signs of something more worrisome. So, we are going to increase my ibuprofen to...not sure I remember the dose, but I know I have to take it four times a day? With food so my stomach doesn't get affected. You are also going to send me to physical therapy."

Provider: "Great! Yes, 600 mg four times a day with food and physical therapy. And we will see each other in 2 weeks." [Provide Closure: Summarize and affirm agreement with the plan of action] "Does that plan seem feasible?" [Reach Agreement on Problems and Plans: Check the patient's willingness and ability to follow the plan]

Patient: "Definitely."

Provider: "And is there anyone you can enlist to help you remember the medication, get to physical therapy, and do more of your physical tasks for you over the next couple of weeks?" [Reach Agreement on Problems and Plans: Identify and enlist resources and supports]

Patient: "My husband has already been a major help, and I could probably enlist my daughter if I need an extra pair of hands."

Provider: "Perfect. What else can I help you with today?" [Provide Closure: Ask whether the patient has other issues or concerns]

Patient: "That's It, Thanks Doc."

MODELS INCORPORATING THE ESSENTIAL ELEMENTS

Conceptual models describe how to approach patient-provider communication in a relationship-centered way. These models bring the essential elements of communication to life.

The Three-Function Model

In 1991, Dr Steven A. Cohen-Cole shared 3 components of the patient interview, which are of critical importance to a successful outcome of the patient-clinician interaction.[15,16] Two of the 3 functions are the traditional core functions of the patient encounter: gather data to understand the patient's problems and educate and motivate the patient to adhere to treatment. The other function of the interview was novel: develop doctor-patient rapport and appropriately respond to patients' emotions.

Rapport is a close, harmonious relationship in which those involved understand each other's feelings or ideas and communicate well. Empathy is the ability to understand and share the feelings of another. Responding appropriately to patients' emotions builds rapport and often requires empathy to be successful. Dr Cohen-Cole identified 5 verbal interventions that serve as a core set of basic skills for this function of developing rapport and appropriately responding to emotions: reflection, legitimation, supportive comments, partnership, and respect (**Fig. 1**).[17]

The principles of the Three-Function Model permeate the Cleveland Clinic REDE to Communicate and Academy of Communication in Healthcare (ACH) Fundamental Skills: RCC models. REDE (Relationship: Establishment, Development and Engagement) is a conceptual framework for teaching and evaluating RCC.[18] The ACH framework similarly identifies 3 groups of skill sets: the encounter beginning, skills that build trust, and delivering diagnoses and treatment plans.[19] These models are available as educational workshops for skills training.

The Structural Model

In 1996, Dr Robert Smith shared the first of now 4 editions of *Patient-Centered Interviewing: An Evidence-Based Method.*[20] This method delineates an 11-step, evidence-based interviewing method to be done sequentially to incorporate patient-centered techniques into the typical provider-patient interview (**Box 3**).

The Structural + Functional Model

The Brown Interview Checklist adopts many of the same principles and attempts to combine both structural and functional approaches by breaking the interview into 2 different sections, namely, the "Flow of the Interview" (akin to the structural model) and "Interpersonal Skills" (akin to the functional model).[15] The flow of the interview includes the opening of the interview, the exploration of problems (or information gathering), and the closing of the interview. Interpersonal skills include facilitation skills and relationship skills, which include all 5 of Cohen-Coles' rapport-building strategies.

The Calgary-Cambridge Guide, introduced by Kurtz and Silverman in 1996, also combines both structural and functional elements of the medical interview.[21] This approach breaks the interview into 6 different domains: initiating the session, gathering information, building a relationship, providing structure, explanation and planning, and closing the visit, inclusive of 12 major steps or items, each composed of multiple microskills.

Finally, the Four Habits model, another evidence-based approach to medical interviewing, combines structural and functional elements.[22] The first and fourth habits, "Invest in the Beginning" and "Invest in the End," are structural in nature. On the other

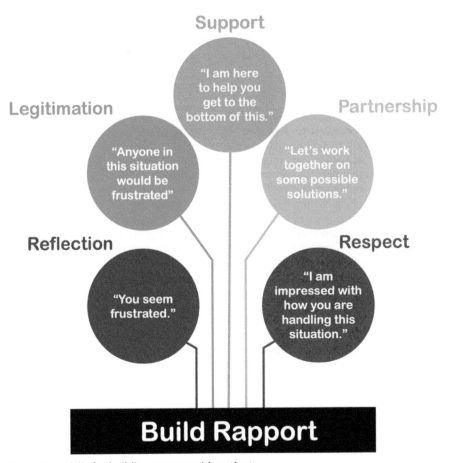

Fig. 1. Core skills for building rapport with patients.

hand, the second and the third habits, "Elicit the Patient's Perspective" and "Demonstrate Empathy," are functionally oriented.

DISCUSSION

Along with the burgeoning patient experience movement, the last 3 decades have given rise to clarity and consensus around the importance of health care communication and the centrality of communication to both patient- and relationship-centered care. Studies have demonstrated a direct link between good communication and outcomes for patients, providers, and institutions. Several models have arisen from the consensus of experts to teach knowledge, skills, and attitudes related to patient-provider communication. Some of these models provide a structural roadmap for the patient interview, whereas others emphasize how communication skills serve different functions in the encounter.

The biggest barriers to implementing relationship-centered care are the lack of provider training in communication and providers' concerns about time. Although most health professions schools now incorporate communication skills training, there are still several generations of physicians in practice who have never received such

---

Box 3
Structural model for patient-provider communication

Step 1: Set the stage for the interview
- Welcome the patient
- Use the patient's name
- Introduce self and identify specific role
- Ensure patient readiness and privacy
- Remove barriers to communication
- Ensure comfort and put the patient at ease

Step 2: Elicit chief concern and set agenda
- Indicate time available
- Forecast what you would like to have happen during the interview
- Obtain list of all issues patient wants to discuss; specific symptoms, requests, expectations, understanding
- Summarize and finalize the agenda; negotiate specifics if too many agenda items

Step 3: Begin the interview with nonfocusing skills that help the patient to express herself/himself
- Start with open-ended request/question
- Use nonfocusing open-ended skills
- Obtain additional data from nonverbal sources: nonverbal cues, physical characteristics, accoutrements, environment, self

Step 4: Use focusing skills to elicit 3 things: symptom story, personal context, and emotional context
- Further elicit symptom story. Description of symptoms, using focusing open-ended skills
- Elicit personal context. Broader personal/psychosocial context of symptoms, patient beliefs/attributions, again using focusing open-ended skills
- Elicit emotional context. Use emotion-seeking skills: direct, indirect, or impact such as belief, triggers, self-disclosure, resonate with unexpressed feeling
- Respond to feelings/emotions. Use empathy skills to address the feelings and emotions such as naming, understanding, respecting, and supporting (NURS)
- Expand the story. Continue eliciting further personal and emotional context; address feelings and emotions (NURS)

Step 5: Transition to middle of the interview
- Brief summary
- Check accuracy
- Indicate that both content and style of enquiry will change if the patient is ready. Continue with middle of the interview.

Step 6: Complete the chronologic description of HPI/OAP

Step 7: Past medical history

Step 8: Social history

Step 9: Family history

Step 10: Review of systems. Continue with physical examination.

Step 11: End of the interview

Reproduced with permission from Fortin VI A, Dwamena F, Frankel R, et al, eds. Smith's patient-centered interviewing: an evidence-based method. 4th edition. McGraw-Hill Companies, Inc.; 2019.

---

training. Several organizations, including the Institute for Healthcare Communication, Cleveland Clinic Foundation, and the Academy of Communication in Healthcare, developed training models for providers in practice. Studies have shown that explicit use of empathic statements can actually shorten visits, and many believe the time gained from anticipating patients' concerns and clarifying misunderstandings around plans more than makes up for any time added by patient-centered skills.[23,24]

SUMMARY

RCC is an effective approach to communicating with patients. Consensus exists regarding the essential elements of communication, and it supports approaching the patient encounter as a set of communication tasks. Building rapport is the most important task. Multiple conceptual models exist, and training in these models can improve a provider's RCC skills.

CLINICS CARE POINTS

- Approach patient communication with the goal of establishing and maintaining a professional relationship.
- Reflect on how you communicate with patients. Do you use the core communication skills, which include empathy, use of open-ended questions, reflective listening, and patient engagement?
- Building rapport is the foundational task of RCC, and it occurs throughout the patient encounter. To build rapport, use the 5 skills that Dr Cohen-Cole delineates.
- Recognize that the conceptual models are not scripts, yet some good habits in communication are worth memorizing.

DISCLOSURE

Drs G. Constant-Peter and R.E. Pearlman are members of the Academy of Communication in Healthcare whose mission is to improve communication and relationships in health care. They are occasionally engaged as consultants and trainers to teach relationship-centered communication.

REFERENCES

1. Stewart M. Towards a global definition of patient centred care: The patient should be the judge of patient centred care. BMJ 2001;322(7284):444–5.
2. Institute of Medicine. Crossing the quality chasm: a new health system for the 21st century 2001. https://doi.org/10.1136/bmj.323.7322.1192.
3. Tresolini, CP and the Pew-Fetzer Task Force. Health Professions Education and Relationship-centered Care. San Francisco, CA: Pew Health Professions Commission; 1994. p. 4–47.
4. Beach MC, Inui T, Frankel R, et al. Relationship-centered care: a constructive reframing. J Gen Intern Med 2006;21(SUPPL. 1). https://doi.org/10.1111/j.1525-1497.2006.00302.x.
5. Aiarzaguena JM, Grandes G, Gaminde I, et al. A randomized controlled clinical trial of a psychosocial and communication intervention carried out by GPs for patients with medically unexplained symptoms. Psychol Med 2007;37(2):283–94.
6. Chassany O, Boureau F, Liard F, et al. Effects of training on general practitioners' management of pain in osteoarthritis: a randomized multicenter study. J Rheumatol 2006;33(9):1827–34. http://www.ncbi.nlm.nih.gov/pubmed/16724375.
7. Girgis A, Cockburn J, Butow P, et al. Improving patient emotional functioning and psychological morbidity: evaluation of a consultation skills training program for oncologists. Patient Educ Couns 2009;77(3):456–62.

8. Bolognesi M, Nigg CR, Massarini M, et al. Reducing obesity indicators through brief physical activity counseling (PACE) in Italian primary care settings. Ann Behav Med 2006;31(2):179–85.

9. Christian JG. Clinic-based support to help overweight patients with type 2 diabetes increase physical activity and lose weight. Arch Intern Med 2008; 168(2):141.

10. Cooper LA, Roter DL, Carson KA, et al. A randomized trial to improve patient-centered care and hypertension control in underserved primary care patients. J Gen Intern Med 2011;26(11):1297–304.

11. Kelley JM, Kraft-Todd G, Schapira L, et al. The influence of the patient-clinician relationship on healthcare outcomes: A systematic review and meta-analysis of randomized controlled trials. PLoS One 2014;9(4).

12. Adams K, Cimino jenica ew, Arnold RM, et al. Why should I talk about emotion? Communication patterns associated with physician discussion of patient expressions of negative emotion in hospital admission encounters. Patient Educ Couns 2012;89(1):44–50.

13. Weiss R, Vittinghoff E, Fang MC, et al. Associations of physician empathy with patient anxiety and ratings of communication in hospital admission encounters. J Hosp Med 2017;12(10):805–10.

14. Participants in the Bayer–Fetzer Conference. Essential Elements of Communication in Medical Encounters. Acad Med 2001;76(4):390–3.

15. Novack DH, Dubé C, Goldstein MG. Teaching medical interviewing. A basic course on interviewing and the physician-patient relationship. Arch Intern Med 1992;152(9):1814–20.

16. Smith M. Book Review: The Medical Interview: The Three-Function Approach. Yale Postgrad Med J 1992;68(799):397–8.

17. Epstein RM, Campbell TL, Cohen-Cole SA, et al. Perspectives on patient-doctor communication. J Fam Pract 1993;37(4):377–88. http://www.ncbi.nlm.nih.gov/pubmed/8409892.

18. Windover AK, Boissy A, Rice TW, et al. The REDE model of healthcare communication: optimizing relationship as a therapeutic agent. J Patient Exp 2014; 1(1):8–13.

19. Academy of Communication in Healthcare. In: Chou C, Cooley L, editors. Communication rx: transforming healthcare through relationship-centered communication. McGraw-Hill Companies, Inc.; 2018.

20. Fortin VIAH, Dwamena FC, Frankel RM, et al, editors. Smith's Patient-Centered Interviewing 4e. 4th edition. McGraw-Hill Companies, Inc.; 2018.

21. Kurtz SM, Silverman JD. The calgary-cambridge referenced observation guides: an aid to defining the curriculum and organizing the teaching in communication training programmes. Med Educ 1996;30(2):83–9.

22. Fossli Jensen B, Gulbrandsen P, Dahl FA, et al. Effectiveness of a short course in clinical communication skills for hospital doctors: results of a crossover randomized controlled trial (ISRCTN22153332). Patient Educ Couns 2011;84(2):163–9.

23. Beach MC, Park J, Han D, et al. Clinician response to patient emotion: impact on subsequent communication and visit length. Ann Fam Med 2021;19(6):515–20.

24. Levinson W, Gorawara-Bhat R, Lamb J. A study of patient clues and physician responses in primary care and surgical settings. JAMA 2000;284(8):1021–7.

25. Rider EA, Nawotniak RH. A Practical Guide to Teaching and Assessing the ACGME Core Competencies. Second Edition. Marbelhead, MA: HCPro, Inc; 2010.

Patient Perspective
Importance and How to Elicit

Mark A. Lewis, MD[a],*, David Bustillo, MS4[b]

KEYWORDS

- Electronic health record • Interpersonal • Communication • Health communication
- Paternalism • Patient preference • Shared decision making

KEY POINTS

- The pendulum has swung away from paternalism toward shared decision making (SDM) as the dominant framework for making medical choices.
- Effective communication between provider and patient results in improved health care outcomes and is positively correlated with patient adherence to therapeutic interventions.
- An important component of effective communication is agenda setting, which aims to prioritize the items to discuss in a visit, a strategy shown to improve patients' health outcomes, satisfaction, and clinician's time management.
- Provider behaviors that promote effective communication include sitting down at the same level of the patient and maintaining eye contact during the interaction.
- The EHR can serve as a repository of information for patients to learn about themselves.

INTRODUCTION

The paradigm guiding interactions between clinician and patient is shifting from paternalism to shared decision making (SDM). In the former model, the formal learning and iterative experience of the doctor are the primary source of therapeutic judgments, but increasingly the patient's embodied perspective is considered when making clinical choices, a shift that respects both an ethical emphasis on autonomy and a pragmatic need to individualize care.[1] Sometimes SDM is contingent upon factors that are known only to the patient and beyond the discernment of quantitative tools at the diagnostician's disposal. Patients are gaining recognition as the "end users" of health care systems, and, as such, their input is being solicited in ways that affect the output of those delivery mechanisms. The challenge arises in where, precisely, to position the locus of control. By virtue of their licensure, physicians must remain the therapeutic effector arm through their ordering privileges, which also protects against the dangers

a Intermountain Healthcare, 5171 S. Cottonwood Street, Building 1, Suite. 610, Murray, UT 84107, USA; b University of California Irvine School of Medicine, 1001 Health Sciences Road, Irvine, CA 92697, USA
* Corresponding author.
E-mail address: mark.lewis2@imail.org

Med Clin N Am 106 (2022) 569–576
https://doi.org/10.1016/j.mcna.2022.01.013
0025-7125/22/© 2022 Elsevier Inc. All rights reserved.

of self-prescription. At the same time, patients understandably wish to retain agency over the decisions that affect their own bodies and outcomes.[2]

HISTORY: THE PAST AS PROLOGUE

Doctors undergo extensive training to benefit their patients by maintaining or restoring their health. Even among modern professionals, this years-long process of learning sets physicians apart from their peers in other fields of doctoral-level study, for example, law, through its rigor and its hierarchical didacticism. In the structure of medical schools and postgraduate residency programs and fellowships, there is an almost anachronistic vestige of guilds whereby apprentices would study under master practitioners to gain specialized understanding.

Historically, the physician's accretion of knowledge and experience was acknowledged with the utmost deference to their judgment, including unilateral determination of care. Within paternalism, the authoritative physician dictates the management of the passive patient. Following the rise of Western liberalism, this model has been rejected as inequitable and unethical in respect to patient autonomy.[3] Other models have been developed in an effort to promote patients' right to self-determination, in turn mandating better communication.

In SDM, each encounter is constructed around mutual respect and participation. Here, the interaction with a health care provider is a collaborative process in which patients gain greater self-understanding and self-determination. Yet, even under the SDM umbrella different approaches exist. In the *informative model*, the clinician provides the patient with all relevant information without recommending a course of action. In the *interpretive model*, the clinician aims to elucidate the patient's values and desires, and to help the patient select the available medical intervention that is most congruent with their principles and goals.[4] Although both models require an explanation beyond the dictums of paternalism, the second is a more open exchange of ideas, a bidirectional discourse that does not presuppose an outcome and calls on both sides to adapt to what they are hearing. This model is particularly well-suited to decisions in which there is more than one medically reasonable option, and the best option hinges on patient preference.[2]

CURRENT EVIDENCE: MAKING THE MOST OF TECHNOLOGY AND TIME IN THE MODERN PATIENT-PHYSICIAN INTERFACE

Of course, there is no *hearing* without *listening*. In her remarkable account as a patient-physician who required critical care after an obstetric catastrophe, Dr Rana Awdish ruefully realizes from her ICU bed that "We [physicians] weren't trained to listen... We were trained to ask questions that steer people to a destination... We weren't trained to value the patient's story."[5]

A conversation requires bilateral engagement and time to talk. Here, the contemporary physician's attention is likely divided, temporally and visually. In a typical outpatient setting, a doctor's work day is organized into blocks, and appointments usually have to conform to an established length, for example, 15 or 30 minutes. Indeed, it is extremely rare, beyond an initial encounter, for an hour to be scheduled for a conversation, even a potentially very difficult and emotionally fraught one like a transition to end-of-life care.

This calendar and its preordained units of time inform the length of each clinic visit, with the doctor aware of how their effort must be allocated for efficient throughput. The patient, however, is likely not cognizant of these time constraints and might perceive their appointment as rushed or their physician as too hurried to attend to their needs.

Observational studies show that physicians tend to interrupt a patient an average of 18 seconds into their presenting complaint[6] and that 50% of psychosocial problems go unaddressed in a usual primary care visit.[7] Time is one of several barriers to developing the patient-clinician relationship (**Box 1**).

Furthermore, the most economical entry of data into the electronic health record (EHR) occurs at the point of care, but this input—if it diverts the physician toward their computer—detracts focus from the very source of information: the patient. Screens and keyboards are nearly omnipresent in examination rooms to enable this midvisit documentation, but "exclusive layouts" can "imped[e] information sharing … and constrai[n] simultaneous data entry and eye contact for clinicians."[8]

For all the sophistication in modern medicine, its core interaction remains the direct encounter between clinician and patient. During the coronavirus disease 2019 (COVID-19) pandemic, some of these have necessarily transitioned from face-to-face visits to virtual platforms. However, the essence of the exchange—a 2-way sharing of information predicated on mutual respect and a sacrosanct commitment to confidentiality—remains intact. The safe conduct of virtual medicine requires stringent standards of cybersecurity, as any data garnered by the clinician is still notated within a firewalled EHR regardless of its source from an in-office appointment, hospital rounds, or virtual consultation. For almost the first time in the history of health care, it is also proof of principle: the locus at which a clinician and their patient meet does not necessarily require shared physical space.

To be sure, there remain tangible and intangible benefits to face-to-face visits; certain provider behaviors can be invaluable in promoting effective communication verbally and nonverbally, including sitting down at the same level and maintaining eye contact during the interaction.[9] If a translator is needed for the patient, then a medically competent interpreter can be provided who is sensitive to the patient's cultural norms and who can provide both "context and information."[10]

As conversations shift to the computer, there is an opportunity to use its platforms as a medium for both parties to communicate, rather than posing a distraction for the clinician-as-scribe. When used to its full potential, the EHR becomes a repository of information not only for health care professionals but also for patients themselves to learn about themselves (**Box 2**). Once again this acknowledges their position at the center of care delivery, because they are the origin and owner of data pertaining to their body. Ideally, patients feel that they are more active participants in their treatment when granted this access.[7]

The "Open Notes" movement embraces transparency and timeliness in the sharing of medical documentation. The near-instantaneous delivery of results through secure patient portals reduces uncertainty and decouples the reporting of a diagnostic test from an in-person visit, potentially enabling asynchronous interaction between the ordering clinician and the patient awaiting results. This eliminates the precarious liminal space of not knowing that Dr Kate Bowler describes as "[building] a home

---

Box 1
Barriers to patient-clinician relationship

- Clinicians may not be properly trained to perceive or value medicine as narrative
- The patient may not be aware of the clinician's time constraints
- Physicians often cannot adjust encounter length to accommodate conversation
- Computers and the electronic health record, if used ineffectively

---

Box 2
Effective ways to use technology for patient empowerment

- Promote MyChart access as a method for patients to learn about themselves
- Decode jargon and provide links to medical glossaries
- Encourage patients to use secure messaging to pose questions to providers

---

[on the side of a cliff]. With each scan, I can feel the upward draft from the deep. And I have to stand however long it takes for a lab tech, two radiologists, then an oncologist, to get back to me and remind me that we have to do this again in a few months."[11]

After years of calls by advocates for immediate access, a proviso of the 21st Century Cures Act—the program rule on Interoperability, Information Blocking, and Office of the National Coordinator (ONC) Health Information Technology Certification—requires that health care providers grant patients the ability to view without charge all the health information in their EHR "without delay." Effective April 5, 2021, the 8 types of clinical notes that must be shared as outlined in the United States Core Data for Interoperability include history and physical, consultation, progress note, discharge summary, imaging narratives, laboratories, pathology reports, and procedure notes. The only exceptions are "psychotherapy notes that are separated from the rest of the individual's medical record and are recorded (in any medium) by a health care provider who is a mental health professional documenting or analyzing the contents of conversation during a private counseling session or a group, joint, or family counseling session" and "information compiled in reasonable anticipation of, or use in a civil, criminal or administrative action or proceeding."[12]

CONTROVERSIES: CHALLENGES IN OBEYING THE SPIRIT OF THE "OPEN NOTES" LAW

Following the legislative charge to grant EHR access to patients, an advocate writing during the law's comment period cautioned that we should not celebrate this digital advance without thinking through its implications on genuine understanding: "Flipping a switch to make notes available does not mean patients are able to find and use them. Truly meaningful efforts… should be the next goal for patients, families and clinicians."[12]

From a technological perspective, the interoperability of EHRs remains an enormous quandary, both between systems and for patients looking to download their data onto their own devices. As such, despite the law taking effect in April 2021, the ONC has allowed until the end of 2022 for implementation and compliance, stating that the Cures Act rule "also aims to increase innovation and competition by fostering an ecosystem of new applications to provide patients with more choices in their healthcare. It calls on the healthcare industry to adopt standardized application programming interfaces (APIs), which will help allow individuals to securely and easily access structured electronic health information using smartphone applications."[13]

Even if the text of notes and reports are rendered immediately available for perusal, the reading comprehension of a lay audience cannot be assumed. George Bernard Shaw wryly observed that the United States and Great Britain are 2 countries divided by a common language; similarly, there are enough differences between conversational English and medical nomenclature that the latter can all too easily lapse into jargon. Critique of the semantics in medicine has even risen to the level of concern that they pose a moral dilemma:

The choice of a particular medical term may deliver different meanings when viewed from these differing perspectives. Consequently, several ethical issues may arise. Technical terms that are not commonly understood by lay people may be used by clinicians, consciously or not, and may obscure the understanding of the situation by lay people. The choice of particular medical terms may be accidental use of jargon, an attempt to ease the communication of psychologically difficult information, or an attempt to justify a preferred course of action and/or to manipulate the decision-making process.[14]

Simply put, the intended "audience" of, say, a radiology report, is a clinician, and the linguistic content of a scan interpretation may need to reimagined with the "patient as end user" in mind. For instance, a patient with cancer might have a radiographically evident tumor variably described as a lesion or mass, with the potential to misinterpret these labels as indicating benignity. Conversely, the incidental finding of, for instance, an adrenal adenoma, pulmonary granuloma, or thyroid nodule may be mistaken for malignancy by a patient who cannot couch those findings in the proper context. Here, asynchronicity impedes patient-clinician communication. If a patient accesses the results of a test when an ordering clinician is unavailable to help them interpret it, the temporal mismatch may engender more apprehension than if the doctor were explaining the clinical meaning in the context of an in-person visit.

APPROACH: FINDING MODERN ANSWERS

Effective communication between provider and patient results in improved health care outcomes[15] and is positively correlated with patient adherence to therapeutic interventions.[7] Clear communication builds and strengthens trust over time,[16] but, by one rubric, only 33% of physicians are considered "excellent" in this domain.[9]

Tai-Seale and colleagues[17] identify an important component of effective communication as "agenda setting, which aims to prioritize the items to discuss in a visit," a strategy shown to "improve patients' health outcomes, satisfaction, and clinician's time management." As such, they developed EHR-based tools to facilitate joint agenda setting as a means of structuring visits in anticipation of and in accordance with mutually identified priorities. A previsit questionnaire was added to the check-in process in the patient-facing EHR portal, prompting them to answer "What is the most important thing you want to discuss with your doctor during your visit?," soliciting a free-form response with a text box allowing up to 250 characters; then, upon that patient's arrival at the appointment, the rooming staff saw a tab in the EHR titled "Patient Important Issues," which also had a documentation shortcut named "PTIMPORTANTISSUES" for prompt incorporation into the clinician's notes.[17] This same process was modified during COVID-19 as a prelude to telehealth visits, demonstrating that it can be adapted to virtual platforms also. Clinician feedback on the addition of this instrument to periappointment workflow largely expressed satisfaction, with comments including "There are no curve balls; I know what the patient wants to talk about before I see them," "It helps them [the patients] focus and get more out of the medical visits," and "The patients listed something that they did not bring up so I was able to ask them about it."[17] For patients returning for annual checkups, it allowed them to narrow the broad generalities of health maintenance and alert their clinician in advance to specific concerns they wanted to address in the limited time together. The investigators conclude that the seamless integration of this prioritization tool into the EHR "could potentially exert a sustained influence on patient and clinician communication behaviors in contrast to prior *ad hoc* educational efforts targeting patients or clinicians."[17]

There are also ongoing efforts to reformat the content of the EHR for better ease of "information consumption" by a broader swath of end users from health care providers to patients themselves. Structured radiology reports, for instance, ensure that all the relevant organs are addressed while also allowing the interpreting physician to relay key findings. Proponents of this format have criticized "traditional narrative reports [as] associated with excessive variability in the language, length, and style, which can minimize report clarity and make it difficult for referring clinicians to identify key information needed for patient care."[18] Eliminating such obfuscation in writing about scans is particularly important if, as mentioned earlier, patients are now granted near-instantaneous electronic access to their own reports.

Finally, humility is the best attitude for the nonpaternalistic physician and is most effective when working *with* patients[17] (**Box 3**). The concept of a team approach, including the patient as an active and valued participant, should be stressed. Explanations should be clear and provided slowly. Among the many tasks of the clinician are to elicit and listen to the stories, opinions, and questions of the patient. The readers can refer to Hofmann and colleagues' article, "Essential Elements of Communication," in this issue for more about relationship-centered communication.

DISCUSSION

An emphasis on interpersonal skills should begin in a practitioner's most formative years, and there have been recent developments in integrating behavioral science and language arts into medical education to cultivate future clinician's ethical mindfulness and emotional capacity.[19,20] However, most training programs do not include communication skills in their curricula.[9] Novel and unforeseeable challenges in care delivery, such as the COVID-19 pandemic, mandate the postgraduate physician's commitment to lifelong learning and adaptation. Flexibility must include adjustment to the changing technologies by which information is relayed to patients and the clinician is cast as an interpreter of data, otherwise threatening to deluge the end user.

Just as necessity is the mother of invention, such new adversities have also given rise to reconception of the patient-clinician interface. Already the pendulum has swung away from paternalism toward SDM as the dominant framework for making medical choices. Now, and in authentic acknowledgment of the patient as a true therapeutic ally in shaping their own care, the adoption of digital tools—spurred on by the pandemic's relocation of some clinical services to virtual platforms—is "leveling the playing field" of medical information by granting both parties access to the EHR. This adoption empowers patients to absorb more data as a means to fuller understand their own health. In the best incarnation of this exchange, patients can express their own priorities to optimize the content and outcome of in-person visits, whereas doctors can plan appointments around foreknowledge of their patients' questions and goals. The once-fallow time between a patient's visits is now a fertile opportunity for further information exchange, including near-immediate delivery of results and anticipation of how emerging facts will reshape understanding and affect future treatment.

Box 3
Clinician-dependent variables valued by patients

- Humility
- Eye contact
- Agenda setting
- Clear and slow explanations

SUMMARY

The dominant paradigm governing patient-physician interaction has shifted from paternalism to SDM. In SDM, information exchange is crucial to allow the provider to understand the patient's preferences and for the patient to make the most educated choices about their own management. Thus, effective communication by doctors may never have been more important than it is now. Key components include agenda setting, clear and slow explanations, eye contact, and humility, of which the last again shifts the locus of control back to the patient in deference to their autonomy. These behaviors demonstrably improve patient satisfaction with their care[21] and authentically embrace the ethos of SDM.

CLINICS CARE POINTS

- Get connected. The EHR can be a superb repository of information by which patients can educate themselves about their medical history.

- Recognize that the data encoded in the EHR may not be clearly understood by lay readers due to formatting and jargon.

- Proactively counsel patients that when they will have access to new test results via electronic portals, such communication is asynchronous and their physicians may not be readily available to help them with real-time interpretation.

DISCLOSURE

No commercial or financial conflicts of interest; no funding sources to declare.

REFERENCES

1. Faiman B, Tariman JD. Shared Decision Making: Improving Patient Outcomes by Understanding the Benefits of and Barriers to Effective Communication. Clin J Oncol Nurs 2019;23(5):540–2. https://doi.org/10.1188/19.CJON.540-542. PMID: 31538972.
2. Kane HL, Halpern MT, Squiers LB, et al. Implementing and evaluating shared decision making in oncology practice. CA Cancer J Clin 2014;64(6):377–88.
3. Chin JJ. Doctor-patient relationship: from medical paternalism to enhanced autonomy. Singapore Med J 2002;43(3):152–5.
4. Emanuel EJ, Emanuel LL. Four models of the physician-patient relationship. JAMA 1992;267(16):2221–6.
5. Awdish R. In Shock: My Journey from Death to Recovery and the Redemptive Power of Hope. Picador; 2018.
6. Groopman J. How doctors Think. Houghton Mifflin; 2007.
7. Stewart MA. Effective physician-patient communication and health outcomes: a review. CMAJ 1995;152(9):1423–33.
8. Zamani Z, Harper EC. Exploring the Effects of Clinical Exam Room Design on Communication, Technology Interaction, and Satisfaction. HERD 2019;12(4): 99–115.
9. Clever SL, Jin L, Levinson W, et al. Does doctor-patient communication affect patient satisfaction with hospital care? Results of an analysis with a novel instrumental variable. Health Serv Res 2008;43(5 Pt 1):1505–19.
10. Rosenblatt A, Kremer M, Paun O, et al. Parental Decision-Making for Surgery and Anesthesia in Young Children. West J Nurs Res 2021. 1939459211021622.

11. Bowler K. No cure for being human. Penguin Random House; 2021.
12. Federal Rules Mandating Open Notes. OpenNotes.org.. Available at: https://www.opennotes.org/onc-federal-rule/. Accessed January 19, 2022.
13. ONC's Cures Act Final Rule. HealthIT.gov.. Available at: https://www.healthit.gov/curesrule/. Accessed January 19, 2022.
14. Shaw D, Manara A, Dalle Ave AL. The ethics of semantics in medicine. J Med Ethics 2021.
15. Zolnierek KB, Dimatteo MR. Physician communication and patient adherence to treatment: a meta-analysis. Med Care 2009;47(8):826–34.
16. Odero A, Pongy M, Chauvel L, et al. Core Values that Influence the Patient-Healthcare Professional Power Dynamic: Steering Interaction towards Partnership. Int J Environ Res Public Health 2020;17(22):8458.
17. Tai-Seale M, Rosen R, Ruo B, et al. Implementation of Patient Engagement Tools in Electronic Health Records to Enhance Patient-Centered Communication: Protocol for Feasibility Evaluation and Preliminary Results. JMIR Res Protoc 2021;10(8):e30431.
18. Ganeshan D, Duong PT, Probyn L, et al. Structured Reporting in Radiology. Acad Radiol 2018;25(1):66–73.
19. Ruberton PM, Huynh HP, Miller TA, et al. The relationship between physician humility, physician-patient communication, and patient health. Patient Educ Couns 2016;99(7):1138–45.
20. Benbassat J, Pilpel D, Tidhar M. Patients' preferences for participation in clinical decision making: a review of published surveys. Behav Med 1998;24(2):81–8.
21. Finefrock D, Patel S, Zodda D, et al. Patient-Centered Communication Behaviors That Correlate With Higher Patient Satisfaction Scores. J Patient Exp 2018;5(3):231–5.

Addressing the Challenges of Cross-Cultural Communication

Carli Zegers, PhD, MBA, APRN, FNP-BC[a],*,
Moises Auron, MD, FAAP, FACP, SFHM[b,c]

KEYWORDS

- Cultural competency • Cultural humility • Cross-cultural communication
- Unconscious biasness • Communication • Cross-cultural • Equity and inclusion
- Health communication

KEY POINTS

- Cross-cultural communication is complex and can be improved with intentional effort and education.
- Cultural humility is a great framework to start improving cross-cultural communication.
- Health communication is directly related to and impacts health, wellness, and equity.
- Training in unconscious bias and communication strategies is a necessary step to improve cross-cultural communication.

INTRODUCTION

Understanding the challenges of cross-cultural communication is critical to improving health and health equity. Traditionally defined, culture is the sum of attitudes, customs, and beliefs that distinguishes one group of people from another.[1,2] Culture is a dynamic integration of complex social and personal elements that are both individually determined and situationally influenced. Culture is also a culmination of interpretation, lived experiences, health beliefs, reactions, and anticipation of future events that create an important focus on time, context, and historical perspectives. The unique attributes of culture manifest differently for each individual and should be celebrated and leveraged in health communication.

[a] University of Kansas, School of Nursing, 3901 Rainbow Boulevard, Mail Stop 4043, Kansas City, KS 66160, USA; [b] Department of Hospital Medicine, Cleveland Clinic Lerner College of Medicine at Case Western Reserve University, Cleveland Clinic, 9500 Euclid Avenue, M2 Annex, Cleveland, OH, USA; [c] Department of Pediatric Hospital Medicine, Cleveland Clinic Lerner College of Medicine at Case Western Reserve University, Cleveland Clinic, 9500 Euclid Avenue, M2 Annex, Cleveland, OH, USA
* Corresponding author.
E-mail address: czegers@kumc.edu
Twitter: @carli_zegers (C.Z.)

Med Clin N Am 106 (2022) 577–588
https://doi.org/10.1016/j.mcna.2022.02.006
0025-7125/22/© 2022 Elsevier Inc. All rights reserved.

A fundamental attribute of culture is language and communication. Communication is a process by which information is exchanged between individuals through a common system of symbols, signs, or behavior.[1,2] Language is a method of communication. Language is defined as words—diction, pronunciation, and methods of combining—that are used and understood by a community. Culture, although expressed through language and communication, is more than shared words, but rather a shared experience. Language and communication in culture is an expression of the shared experience and connects individuals. Cross-cultural communication is often challenging due to the unfamiliar; unfamiliar tone, content, context, preference, or intention. Communication is an exchange of common understanding, and with discordance, there is natural hesitation. Acknowledging communication differences and understanding preferences is very important, especially in medicine.[1,2]

APPROACH AND APPLICATION

A proxy for overcoming challenges of cross-cultural communication is cultural humility. Cultural humility is the art and science developed by Drs Tervalon and Murry-García.[3] Cultural humility is a method of being which incorporates self-evaluation and critique, addresses and redresses power imbalances, and develops mutually beneficial partnerships through a lens of humility.[3] Cultural humility implements self-reflection and awareness as a method to address biases and improves communication. Cultural humility methods allow for improved cross-cultural communication and provide the framework to care for anyone from any culture.

Cultural humility also addresses the limitations of cultural competence. Cultural competence refers to applying knowledge about individuals and groups of people to specific standards, policies, practices, and attitudes.[4] Cultural competence is important for a baseline understanding of different cultural norms and allows for the assessment of knowledge about cultural tendencies. Competence is limited because proficiency is not implementation-focused, but rather serves as a knowledge check. Cultural humility is a dynamic, evolving process and does not have a discrete endpoint like cultural competence.[3] Cultural humility is a skill base and permits cross-cultural communication with all people. **Box 1** describes principles of both cultural humility and cultural competence.

Box 1
Characteristics of cultural competence and humility

Cultural Competence[4]
- Defines culture broadly
- Equates to mastery of an endpoint of understanding
- Is technical and specific to the status quo of current defined culture
- Is community-defining and addresses needs, including language and service
- Institutional-level cultural competence includes staff hiring and training

Cultural Humility[3]
- Requires commitment to lifelong self-evaluation, self-critique, and evolution as a learner
- Encourages redressing power imbalances
- Paves a path to equity
- Supports the development of mutually beneficial, authentic, and respectful partnerships
- Institutional-level cultural humility integrates and develops practices that are flexible and dynamic

Foundational to this framework is the value of humility; an individual will never fully understand another individual entirely, and therefore must mutually respect others' truths and honor dynamic partnerships.[3] The framework allows for individual people to disclose their culture and thus attempts to eliminate assumptions and bias. The premise of cultural humility is that individuals are complex and have intersecting cultural identities that are expressed not as a prescriptive set of rules, but rather are individualized. The limitations of placing individuals within the bounds of a culture are that everyone may manifest their expression and experience differently.[3] An example includes generation variance from religious practices or language. It is important for individuals, institutions, and systems in health care to invest in understanding, implementing, and ensuring cultural humility becomes common practice to improve cross-cultural communication.

Culture influences health in many ways including customs, traditions, celebrations, and lifestyle expectations.[1,2] In addition to understanding language and communication, it is equally important to understand and complement culture-based health preferences and choices. Every person has a culture and experiences it differently. The key is to apply these principles to every patient and ensure that incorporating culture into care is common practice.

Communication, culture, and health intersect at a point of equity. Communication impacts health equity as the current health care system, broadly, relies heavily on patients understanding their health and interacting with the system for use. The Centers for Disease Control and Prevention (CDC) recommends the use of framing both health disparities and public health implications with a health equity lens.[5] The health equity lens allows us to address long-standing inequities by improving policies at all levels and ensuring equitable changes in system-based practice.

As practitioners, understanding and practicing health communication is important to providing health equity at the individual, community, and system levels. On multiple levels, health policy needs to target how discrimination and racism impact and unfairly disadvantage people, especially from historically marginalized groups.[5] Additionally, communicating to ensure patient understanding is essential. Effective cross-cultural communication is not simply ensuring access, but requires more specific and intentional efforts that include engaging individuals from each community. The CDC recommends improving accessibility of content through alternative communication formats and the use of language-specific materials. Most importantly, the CDC recommends that health care via public health programs, policies, and practices should "recognize and reflect the diversity of the community."[5] Addressing cross-cultural communication at this intersection with health is critical to improving health equity and decreasing health disparities. Individual professionals can make a difference by being informed, integrating health equity into practice, and promoting this best practice at institutional and community levels.

NATURE OF THE PROBLEM
Language and Communication in Context

The use of language is extremely important; words, how they are used, and what they mean matter. The variation of language creates connection, and mismatch of communication is a challenge. There are 2 specific examples that demonstrate the unique variability of communication as it relates to culture: code-switching and the Hispanic paradox.

Code-switching is switching from the linguistic system of one language or its dialect to that of another, or "the practice of shifting the languages you use or the way you express yourself in your conversations."[6] Code-switching uses culture to modify language including the use of words, tones, accents, or dialects. Thompson studied reasons to code-switch and identified the top 5 reasons.[6] First, it is natural for people to speak and communicate in the way they were raised so it is inadvert at times. Second, the use of code-switching is to "fit in" as it is a way to connect with others. Next, it serves to actively engage and integrate with others. Fourth, it conveys information as a secret or with hidden meanings.[6] Finally, code-switching allows individuals to better convey a thought through improved expression and word choice as not all languages have words or phrasing that match. Historically, code-switching was used to connect and share identity as the fundamentals of this language type are transforming and borrowing words.[7] The practice of code-switching establishes in-group and out-group language varieties and allows others to connect via language type. Using specific language and code-switching informs and influences social identities and often can reflect "us" versus "them" connections.[7] Code-switching is a way to build trust, engage with others, and understand a complex situation. Therefore, it is important to recognize that variations of language and dialect exist, even in the same language. Such variation is a form of cross-cultural communication. Because language is dynamic and often has variations in meaning, it is important to ensure understanding and partnership with patients.

The next example of the use of language is the Hispanic paradox. The Hispanic paradox is a situation whereby despite expected health trends, Hispanic or Latino individuals have lower mortality rates, especially with cardiovascular disease, than their non-Hispanic/Latino White counterparts. Lower mortality rates are despite all socioeconomic and systemic disparities to which Hispanic individuals are subjected.[8] Although this concept has been studied for more than 30 years, the reason behind this unique paradox is still not completely known, but is often attributed to resiliency through social support and optimism offsetting stress.[9] A strong argument has been made to attribute the positive health status of Hispanics to language. Spanish language is strongly impacted by social connections and strongly associated with self-reported health. Language influences experiences, emotions, and therefore stress appraisal. Coping and stress perception are impacted through contextual factors such as language and culture.[10] As language is the single distinguishing feature of the individuals in this paradox, it must be contributing to stress management and therefore decreasing cardiovascular disease. The 2 proposed pathways include either language directly influences the construction of emotion and the ability to process and manage stress, or Spanish influences cultural practices for social connectedness, emotion, and optimism.[10] Most important is the clear evidence of language and culture on health. Both code-switching and the Hispanic paradox demonstrate the complexity and depth of language and communication, and how important it is to understand the nuances of a patients' language and communication.

Culturally and Linguistically Appropriate Services Standards

To understand the barriers of cross-cultural communication, we must review, understand, and re-envision current policies and standards around communication. The Culturally and Linguistically Appropriate Services (CLAS) standards are fundamental to the discussion of communication (**Table 1**).[11,12] The principal standard is to provide "effective equitable, understandable, and respectful quality care and services that are responsive to diverse cultural health beliefs and practices, preferred languages, health literacy, and other communication needs."[11,12] Adapting these standards is critical for individuals and organizations to improve health equity through communication and provides a "blueprint" for improving cross-cultural communication and care.[11,12]

Table 1
CLAS standards

Principle Standard	Governance, Leadership, and Workforce	Communication Language Assistance	Engagement, Continuous Improvement, and Accountability
• Provide effective equitable, understandable, and respectful quality care and services that are responsive to diverse cultural health beliefs and practices, preferred languages, health literacy, and other communication needs • Example: ensure understanding by using teach-back methods with an interpreter for optimal cross-cultural communication	• Organizational and leadership promote standards including training and integration into policies and practices • Example: review all policies and training on an annual basis	• Ensure language assistance is available and used in every situation without stigma including print and multimedia materials • Example: have American Sign Language readily available and do not use untrained individuals or children for interpreters	• Establish, plan, and integrate organizational goals, policies, and standards that align with CLAS-related activities and measures, including regular assessments of community assets and needs • Example: Set measurable and sustainable goals and expectations including evaluation for all areas of an organization

Use of CLAS standards should be a baseline expectation for all providers, institutions, and systems.

CURRENT EVIDENCE
Destigmatizing Care Intentionally

Globalization and the use of the Internet and social media are catalysts for enhanced awareness of different cultures, professions, lifestyles, art, literature, music genres, and the like. In addition, a rich interaction of diverse people-different nationalities, religions, beliefs, and cultures has become a more common situation in the past century.[13,14] Although bias is a likely inherent characteristic of all civilizations, cross-cultural interactions may be a strong predisposing factor for the expression of bias. All health care providers should receive formal and proper education to create knowledge and awareness around the diversity of cultures, including their own individual expression; in addition, education and development of awareness of conscious or unconscious bias are fundamental.

Awareness of one's own bias is very relevant to the individual physician, as it allows self-reflection. It also becomes a meaningful foundation for the individual to develop more inclusive and respectful communication in cross-cultural interactions. This awareness leads to meaningful efforts to reframe ideas and messages in a different tone and context without losing the original intent, but with inclusion and respect. It also allows providers to pause and enhance clarity in communication with patients.[15]

When patients and colleagues perceive a clinician's genuinely respectful approach to others and witness clear communication, cross-cultural communication is enhanced. This elicits a positive response from any person from any background. This has even been translated into scientific writing, whereby rules to represent race and ethnicity in a clinically relevant and unbiased way are outlined.[16]

The Institute of Medicine has a framework to deliver high value and quality care, which includes 6 aims for the health care system: safe, effective, patient-centered, timely, efficient, and equitable.[17] From these, for the purpose of enhancing communication and respectful interactions with patients, health care should be:

- Patient-centered: Providing care that is respectful of and responsive to individual patient preferences, needs, and values and ensuring that patient values guide all clinical decisions.
- Equitable: Providing care that does not vary in quality because of personal characteristics such as gender, ethnicity, geographic location, and socioeconomic status.

Recently, robust efforts have begun in specific communities, such as using proper pronouns for sexual and gender minority (SGM) persons. This leads to increased confidence to interact in a safe manner with other people without bias. All health care professionals need a strong awareness of these efforts to empower patients, as well as to enhance advocacy toward these communities.[18,19]

In a similar manner, the use of adjectives when referring to patients in oral case presentations impacts bias toward patients. For example, it is not the same to approach a presentation as "50-year-old Black, obese and diabetic man admitted with shortness of breath; he is a smoker…" rather than "50-year-old man admitted with shortness of breath. His past medical history is remarkable for diabetes, obesity and tobacco use (smoking)." In the second presentation, his race was omitted as it does not have a meaningful contribution to the patient's clinical presentation nor to the medical decision making.[20–22] Conscious awareness of this presumably subtle element in a presentation may tremendously impact reframing the content and delivery of the presentation. There is typically no conscious desire to stigmatize patients or have judgment. However, the lack of perception on the contents of the presentation of a clinical case as well as the way the presentation is delivered can negatively impact health care delivery.

In regards to equity, adding social elements such as sexual orientation to a clinical presentation is necessary when this information has implications for clinical decision making. This is relevant as it can enhance the effectiveness of health care delivery in a specific and vulnerable patient population.

Health care communication and medical decision making must also steer away from racial bias. For example, racial bias should not be a barrier to adequate symptomatic and palliative treatments. We must avoid assuming that a patient of a certain ethnic or cultural background will have a higher pain tolerance. Consider sickle cell disease which is common among racial minorities. For a patient with sickle cell crisis, we must limit racial and other implicit bias, provide adequate and appropriate pain control and avoid dismissing the pain as a symptom of opiate dependence.[23]

Resources such as the Implicit Association Test (IAT) are readily available for health care providers, and permit us to reflect and create awareness of unconscious bias. This awareness supports individual efforts to mitigate these biases, positively impacts relationships we have with others from different backgrounds, and promotes more equity, diversity, and inclusion.[23]

Communication challenges arise when treating patients in urban, safety-net hospitals in communities with high levels of violence and crime, and thus high levels of patients with traumatic injuries. The emergency room and hospital teams must remain open in their communication and avoid judgmental attitudes toward patients based on complex and challenging psychosocial backgrounds. For instance, consider taking care of a patient who is a member of an organization characterized by racial discrimination and crimes. Providers can acknowledge that a tattooed symbol relates to that background, but we must also consider the complex psychosocial elements that surround the patient during their lifetime. We may not have awareness of the stressors and situations that each person has experienced during their lifetime that led them to pursue certain behaviors and health risks. Providing empathic, nonjudgmental care often leads to enhanced trust by the patient in the health care system, and may even be a catalyst for patients with challenging backgrounds for positive change in their lives.[24,25] Such cross-cultural communication must remain respectful, neutral, and nonjudgmental, and must focus on the patient's wellness and psychological safety. Intentionally eliminating hate and racial disparities allow for more effective communication and health care delivery.

Eliminate the "Type" of Person as Wrong

As stated in the above section, we must remain neutral to the patient's background or appearance. Certainly, considering the psychosocial elements that may influence the patient's illness is appropriate. Meanwhile, it must not incline the balance toward a bias that can interfere with both health care delivery and its quality.

Patients can have a physical appearance that is dissonant with the provider's cultural background. For example, the presence of a teardrop tattoo may suggest a history of the patient having committed murder in the past. Perhaps that's not the reason for the tattoo. The rationale for having any tattoo is rarely clinically relevant. We must ignore the rationale for this patient to have the tattoo. Being neutral and avoiding premature closure on conclusions about another person is very important. Our privilege to serve and aim to heal must take priority, and avoiding barriers to care simply based on a patient's appearance or background is paramount.[26–28]

Other situations warrant our respect for patient values. Consider a patient with critical illness who is in a very tenuous situation with severe anemia that requires a transfusion, yet the patient does not accept blood as a therapeutic option. We must remain open and respectful, and be creative in implementing a variety of strategies to increase hematopoiesis, achieve hemostasis, and minimize blood loss. Aiming to "convince" patients otherwise would be disrespectful of patient autonomy.[29,30]

Take another patient who has reassigned their gender identity and express this identity. Transgender persons are a minority and face discrimination by society, and sometimes consciously or unconsciously by providers as well. Our degree of comfort in caring for a transgender patient arises from accepting their individuality and again recognizing the privilege we have to be able to care for them. The health care team must focus on the patient as a person. Effective, nonjudgmental communication is a must.[31]

Elevate the Patient

In communication with and about patients, we must maintain neutrality among the different backgrounds, personalities, and self-expressions that our patients manifest, and aim to elevate the patient, placing them in a positive light. This carries tremendous importance in motivational interviewing. Being positive creates a context that allows the patient to reflect and gain insight into their own opportunities for improvement. Positive communication includes acknowledging patient emotions and not avoiding the emotions just to avoid difficult topics.

Considerations
Social determinants of health are fundamental, and we can't ignore their impact on the patient's overall physical and psychological health. The documentation and

presentation of a patient's History and Physical or daily progress in the wards should focus on the meaningful aspects that will impact health care and medical decision making. Documentation and presentations should avoid the use of adjectives or mention of social aspects that can contribute negatively to the perception of the patient, as well as potentially create new barriers to care. However, when these social aspects are relevant to prognosis and the patient's ability to receive treatment, then these must be communicated in a clear, objective, and nonjudgmental way.[32–34]

Providers must be sensitive to the patient's overall socioeconomic status when it comes to determining their ability to effectively receive a treatment. For example, an oral anticoagulant for pulmonary embolism can be prescribed with the rapid discharge of the patient from the hospital. However, if the patient is not able to afford the medication, it is a poor medical decision.[35] If another patient needs dressing changes for a complex wound, but they live in a homeless shelter, we may be biased and assume that appropriate care can't happen in a shelter. However, we may explore along with the social worker whether the shelter would be able to effectively accommodate the patient, or rather continue the patient's care in the hospital until a reasonable and safe discharge is possible.[36,37] In a similar vein, we should be careful when suspecting that patients will not be able to receive proper care at home after a complex hospitalization; unfortunately, such bias has led to a large number of patients to be discharged to skilled nursing facilities.[38] Having a growth mindset and an open and curious approach to overall social and postdischarge resources allows us to make decisions that positively impact the patient's prognosis, well-being, and satisfaction. The open mindset and curiosity also have a strong role in end-of-life care.[39]

DISCUSSION

Overcoming barriers to any challenge first begins with the recognition of the problem. Currently, our system is not yet adequately designed to educate, evaluate, and correct inadequate, deficient, or flippant cross-cultural communication standards or practices. Our system requires a more robust opportunity for culture to be welcomed and supported. Such opportunities rest in the cultural humility elements of life-long learning and continual pursuit of improving self-awareness as health care providers. These principles call for additional work toward improvement, more than just annual modules and single, one-off training.

Training in communication assists efforts to improve cross-cultural communication. There are multiple training options available, including Academy of Communication in Healthcare Relationship-Centered Communication training, motivational interviewing training, and the Clinician Experience Project by Practicing Excellence.[40] Training programs are essential to developing communication skills and becoming more proficient in cross-cultural communication. When deciding on a program, it is important to consider cultural humility elements and ensure the training has a health equity lens.

RECOMMENDATIONS

Challenges in communication have developed in response to complex changes evoked by globalization and enhanced cross-cultural interactions. This has led to the confrontation of different perspectives and cultural backgrounds. Our role in health care is to promote a respectful human coexistence, and living in harmony requires formal awareness of one's own perspective and unconscious bias. Health care providers must ideally reconcile these differences and focus on understanding and embracing their oath in medicine to care for all.[41]

We must be aware that culturally congruent care alone may not be sufficient for effective, inclusive communication. Cultural congruency should not be limited to health care delivery by persons of similar appearance, but also should promote health care teams from all different backgrounds to take care of all persons, regardless of their ethnic, cultural, religious, or social identity. Diversity in health care teams should be promoted and enhanced as this will lead to a more meaningful ability to provide inclusivity and equity in health care delivery.[42] Certainly, the recent challenges of the COVID-19 pandemic have highlighted the importance of cultural congruence in the health care setting.[43]

In addition to the increased diversity in health care providers, the promotion of increased diversity in leadership roles is fundamental, including participation in health care policy creation and implementation to enhance the value of shared decisions across the cross-cultural continuum. It is important to be cognizant of challenges that persons of certain cultures may experience, including discrimination based on gender identity, ethnicity, religion, or country background. We recommend taking this awareness of barriers and enhancing health equity by actively removing such barriers when forming health care teams and caring for patients.

Destigmatizing care is also important. Patient-specific factors such as the patient's race are important to communicate only if its consideration is relevant and contributes meaningfully to patient care.

SUMMARY

In conclusion, there are many challenges when addressing cross-cultural communication. Although there is work involved, addressing these challenges with the strategies outlined is important in decreasing health inequities and improving the health and wellness of our patients. Every person in health care must begin by working on themselves through reflection, intentional practice, and addressing any gaps such as biases. Using the cultural humility framework and working on the unconscious bias are 2 strategies to address such challenges. Additionally, being intentional and mindful of language and important cultural aspects of language helps to appreciate culture and communication as valuable patient attributes. Making efforts at the individual, institutional, and system levels to address cross-cultural communication is essential to creating a more just and equitable health care system.

CLINICS CARE POINTS

- When faced with a cross-cultural communication challenge, use the cultural humility framework to promote culture as an asset rather than a barrier
- When communicating with a patient of a different culture, recognize that culture is complex, and avoid stigmatizing and making assumptions
- To improve cross-cultural communication, pursue intentional training such as unconscious bias and communication techniques training
- When addressing cross-cultural communication at the institutional or health care system level, focus on improving health equity through improving policy and practice. Avoid assuming that a one-time training session is sufficient.
- Recognize that such system-based efforts include institutional and systematic culture shifts to overcome challenges

DISCLOSURE

Dr C. Zegers is a board member of the Academy of Communication in Healthcare whose mission is to improve communication and relationships in health care. She is occasionally engaged as a consultant and trainer to teach relationship-centered communication.

REFERENCES

1. Institute of Medicine (US). Committee on health literacy. In: Nielsen-Bohlman L, Panzer AM, Kindig DA, editors. Health literacy: a prescription to end confusion. Washington, DC: National Academies Press (US); 2004. 4, Culture and Society. Available at: https://www.ncbi.nlm.nih.gov/books/NBK216037/. Accessed October 1, 2021.
2. Culture & health literacy. Centers for Disease Control and Prevention. 2021. Available at: https://www.cdc.gov/healthliteracy/culture.html. Accessed October 3, 2021.
3. Tervalon M, Murray-García J. Cultural humility versus cultural competence: a critical distinction in defining physician training outcomes in multicultural education. J Health Care Poor Underserved 1998;9(2):117–25.
4. "Cultural competence in health and human services." Centers for Disease Control and Prevention, Centers for Disease Control and Prevention. Available at: https://npin.cdc.gov/pages/cultural-competence#3. Accessed October 1, 2021.
5. Using a health equity lens. Centers for Disease Control and Prevention. 2021. Available at: https://www.cdc.gov/healthcommunication/Health_Equity_Lens.html. Accessed September 28, 2021.
6. Thompson M. Five reasons why people code-switch. NPR. 2013. Available at: https://www.npr.org/sections/codeswitch/2013/04/13/177126294/five-reasons-why-people-code-switch. Accessed October 2, 2021.
7. Tannen D, Hamilton HE, Schiffrin D. The handbook of discourse analysis. Malden (MA): John Wiley & Sons, Inc.; 2015.
8. Ruiz JM, Hamann HA, Mehl MR, et al. The Hispanic health paradox: From epidemiological phenomenon to contribution opportunities for psychological science. Group Process Intergroup Relations 2016;19(4):462–76.
9. Gallo LC, Penedo FJ, Espinosa de los Monteros K, et al. Resiliency in the face of disadvantage: do hispanic cultural characteristics protect health outcomes? J Pers 2009;77(6):1707–46.
10. Llabre MM. Insight into the hispanic paradox: the language hypothesis. Perspect Psychol Sci 2021. https://doi.org/10.1177/1745691620968765.
11. Barksdale CL, Rodick WH, Hopson R, et al. Literature review of the national clas standards: Policy and practical implications in reducing health disparities. J Racial Ethn Health Disparities 2016;4(4):632–47.
12. MinorityHealth. Culturally and linguistically appropriate services. Think cultural health. Available at: https://thinkculturalhealth.hhs.gov/clas. Accessed October 1, 2021.
13. Hong YY, Cheon BK. How does culture matter in the face of globalization? Perspect Psychol Sci 2017;12(5):810–23.
14. Yang XL, Liu L, Shi YY, et al. The relationship between cultural anxiety and ethnic essentialism: the mediating role of an endorsement of multicultural ideology. PLoS One 2015;10(11):e0141875.

15. White AA 3rd, Logghe HJ, Goodenough DA, et al. Self-awareness and cultural identity as an effort to reduce bias in medicine. J Racial Ethn Health Disparities 2018;5(1):34–49.

16. Flanagin A, Frey T, Christiansen SL. AMA manual of style committee. Updated guidance on the reporting of race and ethnicity in medical and science journals. JAMA 2021;326(7):621–7.

17. Shenoy A. Patient safety from the perspective of quality management frameworks: a review. Patient Saf Surg 2021;15(1):12.

18. Tavits M, Pérez EO. Language influences mass opinion toward gender and LGBT equality. Proc Natl Acad Sci U S A 2019;116(34):16781–6.

19. Morris M, Cooper RL, Ramesh A, et al. Training to reduce LGBTQ-related bias among medical, nursing, and dental students and providers: a systematic review. BMC Med Educ 2019;19(1):325.

20. Van Ryn M. Avoiding unintended bias: strategies for providing more equitable health care. Minn Med 2016;99(2):40–3.

21. Welch TR, Brown AC, Botash AS. Using student reflective narratives to teach professionalism and systems-based practice. J Pediatr 2017;187:5–6.e1.

22. FitzGerald C, Hurst S. Implicit bias in healthcare professionals: a systematic review. BMC Med Ethics 2017;18(1):19.

23. Hoffman KM, Trawalter S, Axt JR, et al. Racial bias in pain assessment and treatment recommendations, and false beliefs about biological differences between blacks and whites. Proc Natl Acad Sci U S A 2016;113(16):4296–301.

24. Singh K, Sivasubramaniam P, Ghuman S, et al. The dilemma of the racist patient. Am J Orthop (Belle Mead NJ) 2015;44(12):E477–9.

25. Paul-Emile K, Smith AK, Lo B, et al. Dealing with racist patients. N Engl J Med 2016;374(8):708–11.

26. Müller CS, Oertel A, Körner R, et al. Socio-epidemiologic aspects and cutaneous side effects of permanent tattoos in Germany - Tattoos are not restricted to a specific social phenotype. Dermatoendocrinol 2016;9(1):e1267080.

27. Broussard KA, Harton HC. Tattoo or taboo? Tattoo stigma and negative attitudes toward tattooed individuals. J Soc Psychol 2018;158(5):521–40.

28. Byard RW. Potential significance of swastika tattoos in a medico-legal setting. Med Sci Law 2021;61(2):118–21.

29. Bock GL. Jehovah's Witnesses and autonomy: honouring the refusal of blood transfusions. J Med Ethics 2012;38(11):652–6.

30. Rajtar M. Relational autonomy, care, and Jehovah's Witnesses in Germany. Bioethics 2018;32(3):184–92.

31. Safer JD, Tangpricha V. Care of the transgender patient. Ann Intern Med 2019; 171(1):ITC1–16.

32. Johnson TJ. Intersection of bias, structural racism, and social determinants with health care inequities. Pediatrics 2020;146(2). https://doi.org/10.1542/peds. 2020-003657.

33. Mohan G, Chattopadhyay S. Cost-effectiveness of leveraging social determinants of health to improve breast, cervical, and colorectal cancer screening: a systematic review. JAMA Oncol 2020;6(9):1434–44.

34. Karran EL, Grant AR, Moseley GL. Low back pain and the social determinants of health: a systematic review and narrative synthesis. Pain 2020;161(11):2476–93.

35. Nathan AS, Geng Z, Dayoub EJ, et al. Racial, ethnic, and socioeconomic inequities in the prescription of direct oral anticoagulants in patients with venous thromboembolism in the United States. Circ Cardiovasc Qual Outcomes 2019; 12(4):e005600.

36. Kay HF, Sathiyakumar V, Archer KR, et al. The homeless orthopaedic trauma patient: follow-up, emergency room usage, and complications. J Orthop Trauma 2014;28(6):e128–32.

37. Merryman MB, Synovec C. Integrated care: provider referrer perceptions of occupational therapy services for homeless adults in an integrated primary care setting. Work 2020;65(2):321–30.

38. Werner RM, Coe NB, Qi M, et al. Patient outcomes after hospital discharge to home with home health care vs to a skilled nursing facility. JAMA Intern Med 2019;179(5):617–23.

39. Rawlings D, Devery K, Poole N. Improving quality in hospital end-of-life care: honest communication, compassion and empathy. BMJ Open Qual 2019;8(2): e000669.

40. Yuson A, et al. Home." practicing excellence. 2021. Available at: https:// practicingexcellence.com/. Accessed October 1, 2021.

41. Holmboe E, Bernabeo E. The 'special obligations' of the modern Hippocratic Oath for 21st century medicine. Med Educ 2014;48(1):87–94.

42. Schim SM, Doorenbos AZ. A three-dimensional model of cultural congruence: framework for intervention. J Soc Work End Life Palliat Care 2010;6(3–4):256–70.

43. Cuellar NG, Aquino E, Dawson MA, et al. Culturally congruent health Care of COVID-19 in minorities in the United States: a clinical practice paper from the national coalition of ethnic minority nurse associations. J Transcult Nurs 2020;31(5): 434–43.

Health Communication and Sexual Orientation, Gender Identity, and Expression

Carl G. Streed Jr, MD, MPH[a,b],*

KEYWORDS

- Clinical encounter • Gender identity • Gender expression • LGBTQIA
- Sexual and gender minorities • Sexual orientation

KEY POINTS

- Recognize the unique obstacles often encountered by lesbian, gay, bisexual, transgender, queer, intersex, and asexual (LGBTQIA) persons and communities.
- Create and foster the patient–clinician relationship with a population that has and continues to face discrimination from health care systems.
- Use language that does not assume patient orientation, gender, or relationship to other persons and allows an open dialogue with patients to address a variety of issues unique to LGBTQIA persons and communities.
- Accept shared responsibility for eliminating disparities and developing systemic interventions to improve the health and well-being of LGBTQIA persons and communities.

INTRODUCTION

An open dialogue built on trust is required to provide competent and compassionate care for patients and communities. It is the responsibility of clinicians and health care leaders to build and rebuild relationships with individual patients and communities and ensure the health care encounter is welcoming. This article will provide an overview of the experiences of sexual and gender minority (SGM) persons in health care (**Box 1**). SGM communities include lesbian, gay, bisexual, transgender, queer, intersex, and asexual (LGBTQIA) persons and include anyone who does not identify as straight or cisgender (**Table 1**). Meeting the health care needs of SGM persons requires an understanding of sexual orientation, gender identity, and expression of both. Additionally, providing a competent and compassionate clinical encounter requires an understanding of the historical, social, and cultural context of SGM persons.

[a] Section of General Internal Medicine, Department of Medicine, Boston University School of Medicine, Boston, MA, USA; [b] Center for Transgender Medicine and Surgery, Boston Medical Center, 801 Massachusetts Avenue, Room 2082, Boston, MA 02118, *USA*
* 801 Massachusetts Avenue, Room 2082, Boston, MA 02118.
E-mail address: cjstreed@bu.edu
Twitter: @cjstreed (C.G.S.)

Med Clin N Am 106 (2022) 589–600
https://doi.org/10.1016/j.mcna.2021.12.005
0025-7125/22/© 2022 Elsevier Inc. All rights reserved.

HISTORY AND BACKGROUND

Although the science of sexuality and gender acknowledges the existence of same-sex attraction since at least the mid-19th century, most clinicians of the time saw this as an abnormality to be cured or resolved.[1,2] Similarly, while the historical record acknowledges the existence of a diversity of gender identities and gender modalities throughout human existence, Western notions of binary, immutable categories for gender and sex have dictated what is "normal" and "allowable" at many points throughout history.[3,4] While health professions have largely moved from pathologizing to acceptance and support of the full diversity of sexual and gender identities,[5,6] more is needed to ensure SGM persons are able to lead healthy lives that allow them to thrive. This requires clinicians to understand the current landscape of SGM health and policy affecting the lives of SGM persons and communities.

EPIDEMIOLOGY AND OUTCOMES

In comparison with heterosexual and cisgender populations, SGM populations have less favorable overall health and higher rates of cardiovascular disease,[7,8] certain cancers,[9–11] exposure to violence,[12–14] and HIV and other sexually transmitted infections.[15,16] Mental health disparities in SGM populations include higher rates of anxiety, depressive symptoms, and suicidality than among their heterosexual and cisgender counterparts. However, because many studies do not include measures of sexual orientation, gender identity, or intersex status, the full magnitude of health disparities and their effects on SGM populations is not well described. The health and well-being of SGM communities are particularly affected by factors such as discrimination, stigma, prejudice, and other social, political, and economic determinants of health.[17]

CONSIDERATIONS: MINORITY STRESS

Individual and institutional discrimination cause direct harm to the well-being of persons and communities.[18] Research demonstrates the harmful effects of discrimination among several marginalized groups including racial and ethnic minority adults.[19,20] The stress of experiencing and facing discrimination and structural inequity based on identity is posited as one the main drivers of health disparities experienced by SGM persons and communities.[7,8,17,21] The predominant theory to explain SGM health disparities is the *minority stress model* (**Fig. 1**) which describes how, in addition to general life stressors we all may face, SGM persons are exposed to minority stressors that contribute to disparities in health outcomes. Originally developed to study mental health disparities in sexual minorities, the minority stress model was later adapted for gender minority health.[8,22] In addition, the *social ecological model*

Box 1
National Institutes of Health definition of sexual and gender minorities[44]

SGM populations include, but are not limited to, individuals who identify as lesbian, gay, bisexual, asexual, transgender, Two-Spirit, queer, and/or intersex. Individuals with same-sex or -gender attractions or behaviors and those with a difference in sex development are also included. These populations also encompass those who do not self-identify with one of these terms but whose sexual orientation, gender identity or expression, or reproductive development is characterized by nonbinary constructs of sexual orientation, gender, and/or sex.

Table 1 Definitions	
Asexual	A Term Used to Describe Someone Who has Little or No Sexual Attraction to Others. Asexual People can Experience Other Forms of Attraction.
Bisexual	Someone who experiences sexual, romantic, physical, and/or spiritual attraction to people of their own gender as well as toward another gender. (sometimes shortened to "bi")
Cisgender	A term used to describe people whose gender identity is congruent with what is traditionally expected based on their sex assigned at birth.
Gay	A term used to describe boys/men who are attracted to boys/men, but often used and embraced by people with other gender identities to describe their same-gender attractions and relationships as well. Often referred to as "homosexual," though this term is no longer used by the number of people with same-gender attractions.
Gender diverse	A term used to describe people whose gender identity is not constrained by binary concepts of gender.
Gender expression	The ways in which a person communicates femininity, masculinity, androgyny, or other aspects of gender, often through speech, mannerisms, gait, or style of dress. Everyone has ways in which they express their gender.
Gender identity	A person's inner sense of being a girl/woman, a boy/man, a combination of girl/woman and boy/man, something else, or having no gender at all. Everyone has a gender identity.
Gender minority	A broad diversity of people who experience an incongruence between their gender identity and what is traditionally expected based on their sex assigned at birth, such as transgender and gender diverse persons.
Gender nonbinary	A term used by some people who identify as a combination of girl/woman and boy/man, as something else, or as having no gender. Often used interchangeably with "gender nonconforming."
Gender nonconforming	A term used by some people who identify as a combination of girl/woman and boy/man, as something else, or as having no gender. Often used interchangeably with "gender nonbinary."
Lesbian	Used to describe girls/women who are attracted to girls/women; applies for cisgender and transgender girls/women. Often referred to as "homosexual," though this term is no longer used by the number of women with same-gender attractions.
Queer	Historically a derogatory term used against LGBTQ people, it has been embraced and reclaimed by LGBTQ communities. Queer is often used to represent all individuals who identify outside of other categories of sexual and gender identity. Queer may also be used by an individual who feels as though other sexual or gender identity labels do not adequately describe their experience.
Sex assigned at birth	Usually based on phenotypic presentation (ie, genitals) of an infant and categorized as women or men; distinct from gender identity.
Sex	Biological sex characteristics (chromosomes, gonads, sex hormones, and/or genitals); men, women, intersex. Synonymous with "sex assigned at birth."

(continued on next page)

Table 1 (continued)	
Sexual minority	A broad diversity of people who have a sexual orientation that is anything other than heterosexual/straight, and typically includes gay, bisexual, lesbian, queer, or something else.
Sexual orientation	A person's physical, emotional, and romantic attachments in relation to gender. Conceptually separate from gender identity and gender expression. Everyone has a sexual orientation.
Straight	A boy/man or girl/woman who is attracted to people of the other binary gender than themselves; can refer to cisgender and transgender individuals. Often referred to as heterosexual.
Transgender man	Someone who identifies as men but was assigned women sex at birth.
Transgender woman	Someone who identifies as women but was assigned men sex at birth.

Adapted from Streed et al. 2021[7].

recognizes how a person's health is influenced by factors in their social environment, such as interpersonal (eg, family, friends), community, and societal factors.[23] **Fig. 1.** General stressors faced by SGM persons and communities include:

- Higher likelihood of reporting physical and sexual abuse in childhood.[24,25]
- Higher prevalence of interpersonal violence in adulthood.[26,27]
- Higher rates of poverty than cisgender heterosexual people (21.6% vs 15.7%) with poverty rates highest among bisexual men (19.5%) and women (29.4%), transgender people (29.4%), and SGM people living in rural areas.[28]

When exploring the intersection of SGM identity with racial and ethnic identities, within the SGM population, Latine (37.3%), Black (30.8%), and American Indian/Native Alaskan (32.4%) adults are more likely to live in poverty compared with their White peers (15.4%).[28]

Minority stressors that relate to SGM status exist at multiple levels with decades of research highlighting the disparities and inequities faced by SGM persons and communities. Data from a 2017 nationally representative, probability-based survey of

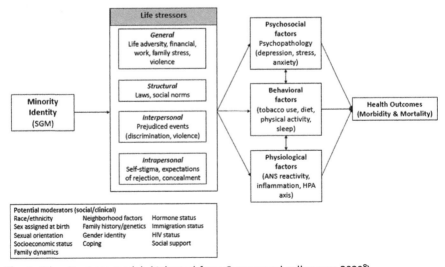

Fig. 1. Minority stress model. (*Adapted from* Caceres and colleagues 2020[8])

more than 3000 adults conducted for National Public Radio, the Robert Wood Johnson Foundation, and Harvard T.H. Chan School of Public Health found that SGM adults reported significant individual and institutional experiences of discrimination, across many aspects of life.[29]

Looking specifically at individual experiences of discrimination, number of all SGM people have experienced slurs (57%) and insensitive or offensive comments (53%) about their sexual orientation or gender identity. Number of LGBTQIA people say that they or an SGM friend or family member have been threatened or nonsexually harassed (57%), been sexually harassed (51%), or experienced violence (51%) because of their sexuality or gender identity. More than a third (34%) of all SGM people say that they or an SGM friend or family member have been verbally harassed in the bathroom or been told or asked if they were using the wrong bathroom.

These experiences of discrimination are part of the larger context of structural discrimination when we examine experiences of institutional discrimination. At least one in five SGM people report being personally discriminated against because of their sexuality or gender identity when applying for jobs (20%), when being paid equally or considered for promotion (22%), or when trying to rent a room or apartment or buy a house (22%). More than a quarter of SGM people say that they or a friend or family member who is also SGM have been unfairly stopped or treated by the police (26%) or unfairly treated by the courts (26%) because they are part of the SGM community.

Perhaps most damning is the experience of discrimination in health care. Roughly one in six SGM people say they have avoided medical care (18%) due to concern that they would be discriminated against because of their SGM identity. One in ten transgender persons reported being personally discriminated against because they are transgender when going to a doctor or health clinic. Over 1 in 5 (22%) transgender persons say they have avoided a doctor or health care out of concern that they would be discriminated against because they are transgender. Nearly a third (31%) of transgender persons reported not having a regular doctor or health care professional that provides most of their health care when sick or having a health concern.

As sexual orientation, gender identity, and expression intersect with other marginalized identities, it is critical to know the experience of SGM persons of color. SGM persons of color are at least twice as likely as white SGM persons to have been personally discriminated against because they are SGM when applying for jobs and when interacting with police.

Specific to the importance of communicating with SGM persons in clinical settings, clinicians must understand the stress associated with incorrect names and pronouns; or rather the power of correctly utilizing a patients' name and pronouns. Data from a community cohort sample of transgender youth from across three U.S. cities found that, after adjusting for personal characteristics and social support, correct name use in more contexts was associated with lower depression, suicidal ideation, and suicidal behavior. Notably, depression, suicidal ideation, and suicidal behavior were lowest when chosen names could be used in all studied contexts.[30] Essentially, for transgender youth who use a name different from the one given at birth, use of their chosen name in multiple contexts affirms their gender identity and reduces mental health risks.

Recognizing the disparate experiences of SGM persons and the ways in which individuals, communities, institutions, and society treats SGM persons is critical to addressing their health and well-being. With Minority Stress Theory as a framework to understand the health of marginalized populations such as SGM persons and communities, we can begin to build a better health care experience and system to meet their unique needs.

APPLICATION
Access

Access to comprehensive, affirming, and high-quality health care services, and laws that guarantee access to health care services, health insurance coverage, and health care for all, regardless of sexual orientation, gender identity, and intersex status, are critical to the health and well-being of SGM persons and communities. As negative experiences with health care are common for SGM persons, they are looking for some indication that their clinical care will be, at minimum, not traumatizing, and, ideally, be competent and compassionate. As such, the ways in which institutions and clinicians signal their inclusion and competency to care for SGM person matters. There are various rating systems for health care institutions to assess their ability to provide competent and compassionate care to SGM persons and communities. The Human Rights Campaign Health Equality Index, for example, offers health care facilities a powerful way to affirm that they comply with Joint Commission and Centers for Medicare and Medicaid Services requirements as well as Section 1557 of the Affordable Care Act (ACA). Designation as a leader on the Health Equality Index also signals to SGM persons that the facility is committed to SGM care.

Further, potential patients will be looking at specific environmental cues in the clinic space, particularly symbols of inclusion. These include diverse representations of relationships in office décor, gender-neutral facilities, and explicit cues that SGM persons are welcome (e.g., rainbow flag).

Intake

The intake process, particularly intake forms, signals the general preparedness of a clinical setting to care for SGM persons. Through intake forms, patients can be given the opportunity to share upfront their correct name, pronouns, sexual orientation, and gender identity. Whenever possible it is best to use open-ended questions; it may be better to offer a blank space for the patient to fill in an answer instead of checkboxes that only offer a limited number of responses.[31,32] **Figs. 2** and **3**.

Despite recommendations to collect sexual orientation and gender identity data and the requirement that electronic health records be capable to collect this data,[33,34] many have not expanded data fields to include all aspects of data relevant to patient care. While provider discomfort is often cited as a reason for low sexual orientation and gender identity data collection,[35,36] all patients report high levels of acceptance and satisfaction when personal sexual orientation and gender identity data are collected.[37] Opportunities for provider training exist through the National Center for LGBT Health Education and the Human Rights Campaign. Additional resources are found in collaboration with local SGM community organizations as well as professional organizations (e.g., American Medical Association, American College of Physicians, and American Academy of Pediatrics). Patients want to provide this information and are comfortable sharing this part of their identity with welcoming clinicians.

Encounter

Once the patient has arrived at a health care institution and navigated the intake process, it is up to the clinical team to ensure the patient has a welcoming experience. Staff should always look at the name and pronoun data prior to interacting with patients to ensure their proper use for the patient. If staff are unsure about names or pronouns, they can simply ask patients politely what they would like to be called and what pronouns they use. Staff can also be trained to address patients in a gender-neutral manner, such as "the patient is in the waiting room," rather than "he/she is in the waiting room."

Demographics Form

Today's Date

____ / ____ / 20____

Name on ID/Insurance: First		Middle	Last		New Patient? Yes No
Chosen First Name:			Birth Date: Month Day Year / /		
Have you attended Outreach Events Yes No		Do you receive public benefits (SNAP, medical card, etc.) Yes No			
Pronouns: ☐ He/him ☐ She/her ☐ They/them ☐ Only my name ☐ No preference ☐ A pronoun not listed ____					

We require the following information for the purposes of helping our staff use the most respectful language when addressing you, understanding our population better, and fulfilling our grant reporting requirements. The options for some of these questions were provided by our funders; we understand that current demographic categories do not adequately capture our individual identities. Please help us serve you better by selecting the best answers to these questions. Thank you.

Fig. 2. Intake form header from Howard Brown Health, Chicago, IL

The clinician leading the encounter must demonstrate competence in welcoming the patient and gathering information in a nonjudgmental, affirming, and open manner (**Table 2**). With every patient encounter, greeting the patient and whoever may be accompanying them sets the tone for the entire visit. The purpose of including complete data collection on intake is to avoid making assumptions about gender identity or sexual orientation. Specifically, the gender identity or sexual orientation of the patient should never be assumed based on name or outward appearances or even name in the medical chart; transgender patients may still be in the process of aligning their legal name with their gender identity. It is, therefore, important that until the patient's pronouns or correct name is known, they should be addressed by their full name, not as "Mr Smith" or "Ms Smith." Further, never presume to know the relationship of anyone accompanying the patient; too often are significant others mistaken for "brother," "sister," or "friend." Making an assumption, no matter how benign and unintentional, can signal to the patient that the health care provider is at best not trained to manage patients with SGM and at worst intolerant or hostile. If the clinician

Gender Identity:

☐ Male/Man

☐ Female/Woman

☐ Trans Male/Trans Man

☐ Trans Female/Trans Woman

☐ Genderqueer/Gender nonconforming

☐ Something else

☐ Decline to answer

Sexual Orientation:

☐ Lesbian ☐ Straight

☐ Gay ☐ Something else

☐ Bisexual ☐ Questioning

☐ Queer ☐ Decline to answer

Sex Assigned at Birth:

☐ Male ☐ Intersex

☐ Female ☐ Decline to answer

Fig. 3. Sexual orientation and gender identity questions on intake form from Howard Brown Health, Chicago, IL

unintentionally makes an assumption, providing an immediate apology often corrects the *faux pas* and can allow the provider and the patient to set the encounter on the right path.

After greetings, introductions, and establishing rapport, the clinical encounter can transition to eliciting the chief concern of the patient. Providing undivided attention and exhibiting interest with nonverbal cues will signal engagement, and maintaining an appropriate level of eye contact will allow the patient to feel more welcome. Too often have patients with SGM been dismissed by providers who looked at the patient with a degree of disgust or judgment or never looked them in the eye (see **Table 2**).

Documentation

Recognizing the individual- and population-level value of sexual orientation and gender identity data collection, the Centers for Medicare & Medicaid Services (CMS) and the Office of the National Coordinator of Health Information Technology require all electronic health record systems certified under Stage 3 of the Meaningful Use program to allow users to record, change, and access structured data on sexual orientation and gender identity.[38,39] Further, the Human Resources Services Administration (HRSA) Bureau of Primary Health Care began requiring federally funded community health centers to collect and provide sexual orientation and gender identity data in 2016 as part of their annual Uniform Data Systems report. However, a secondary analysis of sexual orientation and gender identity data collection from 2016 reported by 1367 US health centers caring for nearly 26 million patients in the U.S. and territories indicates disappointing uptake of sexual orientation and gender identity data collection. Over three-quarters (77.1%) of patients did not have sexual orientation and gender identity status documented in their electronic health records.[40] The delay in proper documentation of sexual orientation, gender identity, name, and pronouns for patients is a failure to meet the needs of SGM persons and communities. Without appropriate data collection and documentation, identifying disparities and addressing the unique needs of SGM persons is made more difficult.

These requirements from HRSA, CMS, and the ACA can motivate the appropriate collection and documentation of sexual orientation and gender identity patient

Table 2 Helpful hints during the clinical encounter	
Use Correct Name	This Should be Addressed on Intake and Noted in all Future Visits
Use Correct Pronouns	This should be addressed on intake and noted in all future visits If pronouns are not known, avoid binary pronouns in documentation
Do Not Make Assumptions About Gender	If the patient notes that they are not single, do not assume the gender of their significant other. Avoid "girlfriend," "boyfriend," "wife," and "husband" unless the patient uses these terms.
Do Not Make Assumptions About Relationships	Do not say, "and is this your sister [brother/mother/father]?" Say, "and who has joined you today?" and allow the companion to identify themselves and their relationship to the patient
Use Open-Ended Questions	Use open-ended questions to elicit information about your patient and their health, behaviors, and social support.

Box 2

Additional resources for sexual orientation and gender identity data collection

- *The Nuts and Bolts of SOGI Data Implementation: A Troubleshooting Toolkit*: https://assets2. hrc.org/files/assets/resources/Implementing_SOGI_Data_Collection_Practices.pdf
- *Ready, Set, Go! A Guide for Collecting Data on Asexual Orientation and Gender Identity*: https://www.lgbtqiahealtheducation.org/wp-content/uploads/2018/03/TFIE-47_Updates-2020-to-Ready-Set-Go-publication_6.29.20.pdf

---

information in the electronic health record. To achieve this, it is necessary to build a coalition of support at your organization and address the various steps of implementation. For many organizations, the implementation of sexual orientation and gender identity data collection can seem like an overwhelming task. Thankfully, there are numerous guides to help facilitate this process and no organization needs re-invent the wheel to meet the needs of SGM persons.[37,41–43] **Box 2**.

DISCUSSION

Given the extensive history of discrimination and abuse experienced by SGM persons when accessing health care, a positive clinical encounter will begin to address the health disparities experienced by SGM communities. To that end, it is also important to be open to feedback from patients with SGM; often they are in a position to educate their providers and have had to do so in the past. Additionally, it is important to note that patients with SGM have long been providing one another referrals to providers that have demonstrated culturally competent and compassionate care; the best referral comes from a satisfied patient. If the encounter has provided for at least the beginning of an open dialogue, patients with SGM will continue to seek care. The more positive encounters that occur between the health care professions and SGM population, the sooner disparities in health care outcomes in patients with SGM will be understood and addressed.

SUMMARY

LGBTQIA persons and communities often encounter unique obstacles in life and continue to face discrimination from health care systems. Clinicians are poised to accept shared responsibility for eliminating disparities and developing systemic interventions to improve the health and well-being of LGBTQIA persons and communities. Creating and fostering the patient–clinician relationship can mitigate challenges. Diction matters, and clinicians should use language that does not assume patient orientation, gender, or relationship to other persons, and that allows an open dialogue to address a variety of issues unique to this population.

CLINICS CARE POINTS

- *Minority Stress Theory* tells us that the way society treats SGM persons affects their health now and in the future
- *Use Correct Name*—do not assume patient's legal name is their correct name
- *Use Correct Pronouns*—use gender-neutral pronouns until the patient indicates otherwise, then use the correct pronoun

- *Do Not Assume Gender*—gender expression and gender identity are related but one does not dictate the other
- *Do Not Make Assumptions About Relationships*—ask about the patient's relationships with other people, who are their support system, and who has accompanied them to the clinical encounter
- *Collect Patient Information*—implement the appropriate collection of sexual orientation, gender, identity, patient name, patient pronouns. Patients want to share this information to improve their clinical care.
- *There Is No Such Thing As "Normal"*—embrace the diversity of sexuality and gender and your practice will be more inclusive

DISCLOSURE

The author has nothing to disclose.

ACKNOWLEDGEMENTS

Streed reports salary support from a National Heart, Lung, and Blood Institute career development grant (NHLBI 1K01HL151902-01A1), an American Heart Association career development grant (AHA 20CDA35320148), the Providence/Boston Center for AIDS Research Interest Group (P30AI042853-23), and the Boston University School of Medicine Department of Medicine Career Investment Award.

REFERENCES

1. Streed CG Jr, Anderson JS, Babits C, et al. Changing medical practice, not patients - putting an end to conversion therapy. N Engl J Med 2019;381(6):500–2.
2. Terry J. An American obsession : science, medicine, and homosexuality in modern society. Chicago, IL: University of Chicago Press; 1999. p. 537, xiv.
3. Manion J. Female husbands: a trans history. Cambridge University Press; 2020.
4. Beemyn G. US history. In: Erickson-Schroth L, editor. Trans bodies, trans selves: a resource for the transgender community. New York, NY: Oxford Univeristy Press; 2014. p. 501–36, chap 22.
5. Slagstad K. The political nature of sex - transgender in the history of medicine. N Engl J Med 2021;384(11):1070–4.
6. American Medical Association. Medical spectrum of gender D-295.312. 2018. https://policysearch.ama-assn.org/policyfinder/detail/spectrum%20gender?uri=%2FAMADoc%2Fdirectives.xml-D-295.312.xml.
7. Streed CG Jr, Beach LB, Caceres BA, et al. Assessing and addressing cardiovascular health in people who are transgender and gender diverse: a scientific statement from the american heart association. Circulation 2021;144(6):e136–48.
8. Caceres BA, Streed CG Jr, Corliss HL, et al. Assessing and addressing cardiovascular health in LGBTQ adults: a scientific statement from the american heart association. Circulation 2020;142(19):e321–32.
9. Boehmer U, Elk R. LGBT populations and cancer: is it an ignored epidemic? LGBT Health 2015. https://doi.org/10.1089/lgbt.2015.0137.
10. Boehmer U, Gereige J, Winter M, et al. Transgender individuals' cancer survivorship: Results of a cross-sectional study. Cancer 2020;126(12):2829–36.
11. Boehmer U, Ozonoff A, Potter J. Sexual minority women's health behaviors and outcomes after breast cancer. LGBT Health 2015;2(3):221–7.

12. Valentine SE, Peitzmeier SM, King DS, et al. Disparities in exposure to intimate partner violence among transgender/gender nonconforming and sexual minority primary care patients. LGBT Health 2017;4(4):260–7.
13. Meyer IH, Luo F, Wilson BDM, et al. Sexual orientation enumeration in state anti-bullying statutes in the United States: associations with bullying, suicidal ideation, and suicide attempts among youth. LGBT Health 2019;6(1):9–14.
14. Bouris A, Everett BG, Heath RD, et al. Effects of victimization and violence on suicidal ideation and behaviors among sexual minority and heterosexual adolescents. LGBT Health 2016;3(2):153–61.
15. Center for Disease Control and Prevention. Estimated HIV incidence and prevalence in the United States 2014–2018. HIV Surveill Supplemental Rep 2020;25(1): 18–34. Available at: https://www.cdc.gov/hiv/pdf/library/reports/surveillance/cdc-hiv-surveillance-supplemental-report-vol-25-1.pdf.
16. Sharma A, Wang LY, Dunville R, et al. HIV and sexually transmitted disease testing behavior among adolescent sexual minority males: analysis of pooled youth risk behavior survey data, 2005-2013. LGBT Health 2017;4(2):130–40.
17. Meyer IH. Resilience in the study of minority stress and health of sexual and gender minorities. Psychol Sex Orientation Gend Divers 2015;2(3):209–13. https://doi.org/10.1037/sgd0000132. Resilience in Minority Stress of Lesbians, Gay Men, Bisexuals and Transgender People.
18. National Academies of Sciences Engineering and Medicine (NASEM). Understanding the well-being of LGBTQI+ populations. Washington, DC: The National Academies Press; 2020.
19. Sims M, Glover LSM, Gebreab SY, et al. Cumulative psychosocial factors are associated with cardiovascular disease risk factors and management among African Americans in the Jackson Heart Study. BMC Public Health 2020;20(1):566.
20. Cavanagh L, Obasi EM. The moderating role of coping style on chronic stress exposure and cardiovascular reactivity among african american emerging adults. Prev Sci 2020;22. https://doi.org/10.1007/s11121-020-01141-3.
21. Meyer IH. Minority stress and mental health in gay men. J Health Soc Behav 1995;36(1):38–56.
22. Testa RJ, Habarth J, Peta J, et al. Development of the gender minority stress and resilience measure. Psychol Sex Orientation Gend Divers 2015;2(1):65–77.
23. McLeroy KR, Bibeau D, Steckler A, et al. An ecological perspective on health promotion programs. Health Educ Q Winter 1988;15(4):351–77.
24. Balsam KF, Rothblum ED, Beauchaine TP. Victimization over the life span: a comparison of lesbian, gay, bisexual, and heterosexual siblings. J Consult Clin Psychol 2005;73(3):477–87.
25. Merrick MT, Ford DC, Ports KA, et al. Prevalence of adverse childhood experiences from the 2011-2014 behavioral risk factor surveillance system in 23 states. JAMA Pediatr 2018;172(11):1038–44.
26. Chen PH, Jacobs A, Rovi SL. Intimate partner violence: IPV in the LGBT community. FP Essent 2013;412:28–35.
27. Ard KL, Makadon HJ. Addressing intimate partner violence in lesbian, gay, bisexual, and transgender patients. J Gen Intern Med 2011;26(8):930–3.
28. Badgett MVL, Choi SK, Wilson BDM. LGBT poverty in the United States: a study of differences between sexual orientation and gender identity groups. Los Angeles, CA: The Williams Institute; 2019. Available at: https://williamsinstitute.law.ucla.edu/wp-content/uploads/National-LGBT-Poverty-Oct-2019.pdf.
29. N.P.R. RWJF, Harvard TH Chan School of Public Health,. Discrimination in America: Experiences and Views of LGBTQ Americans. 2017. November 2017.

Available at: https://cdn1.sph.harvard.edu/wp-content/uploads/sites/94/2017/11/NPR-RWJF-HSPH-Discrimination-LGBTQ-Final-Report.pdf. Accessed December 18, 2019.

30. Russell ST, Pollitt AM, Li G, et al. Chosen name use is linked to reduced depressive symptoms, suicidal ideation, and suicidal behavior among transgender youth. J Adolesc Health 2018;63(4):503–5.

31. The Joint Commission. Advancing effective communication, cultureal competence, and patient- and famly-centered care for the lesbian, gay, bisexual, and transgender (LGBT) community: a field guide. Washington, DC: The Joint Commission; 2011. Available at: http://www.jointcommission.org/assets/1/18/LGBTFieldGuide.pdf.

32. The Joint Commission. Collecting sexual orientation and gender identity data in electronic health records: workshop summary. 2013. Available at: http://www.ncbi.nlm.nih.gov/pubmed/23967501. Accessed December 10, 2017.

33. Streed CG Jr, Grasso C, Reisner SL, et al. Sexual orientation and gender identity data collection: clinical and public health importance. Am J Public Health 2020; 110(7):991–3.

34. Baker KE, Streed CG, Durso LE. Ensuring that LGBTQI+ people count — collecting data on sexual orientation, gender identity, and intersex status. N Engl J Med 2021;384(13):1184–6.

35. Haider AH, Schneider EB, Kodadek LM, et al. Emergency department query for patient-centered approaches to sexual orientation and gender identity : the equality study. JAMA Intern Med 2017;177(6):819–28.

36. Haider A, Adler RR, Schneider E, et al. Assessment of patient-centered approaches to collect sexual orientation and gender identity information in the emergency department: the equality study. JAMA Netw Open 2018;1(8):e186506.

37. Cahill S, Singal R, Grasso C, et al. Do ask, do tell: high levels of acceptability by patients of routine collection of sexual orientation and gender identity data in four diverse American community health centers. PLoS One 2014;9(9):e107104.

38. 42 CFR Parts 412 and 495 [CMS-3310-FC and CMS-3311-FC], RINs 0938-AS26 and 0938-AS58. Medicare and Medicaid Programs; Electronic Health Record Incentive Program—Stage 3 and Modifications to Meaningful Use in 2015 through 2017. (2015).

39. Cahill SR, Baker K, Deutsch MB, et al. Inclusion of sexual orientation and gender identity in stage 3 meaningful use guidelines: a huge step forward for LGBT health. LGBT Health 2016;3(2):100–2.

40. Grasso C, Goldhammer H, Funk D, et al. Required sexual orientation and gender identity reporting by us health centers: first-year data. Am J Public Health 2019;e1–8.

41. Suen LW, Lunn MR, Katuzny K, et al. What sexual and gender minority people want researchers to know about sexual orientation and gender identity questions: a qualitative study. Arch Sex Behav 2020;49(7):2301–18.

42. Rullo JE, Foxen JL, Griffin JM, et al. Patient acceptance of sexual orientation and gender identity questions on intake forms in outpatient clinics: a pragmatic randomized multisite trial. Health Serv Res 2018;53(5):3790–808.

43. Morgan R, Dragon C, Daus G, et al. Updates on Terminology of sexual orientation and gender identity survey measures. FCSM 20-03. Federal committee on statistical methodology. Available at: https://nces.ed.gov/fcsm/pdf/FCSM_SOGI_Terminology_FY20_Report_FINAL.pdf. Accessed October 25, 2020.

44. Sexual and gender minority populations in NIH-supported research NOT-OD-19-139. National Institutes of Health); 2019.

The Diagnostic Medical Interview

Jessica J. Dreicer, MD[a,*], Andrew S. Parsons, MD, MPH[a], Joseph Rencic, MD[b]

KEYWORDS

- History-taking • Diagnosis • Medical interview • Clinical reasoning
- Health care communication

KEY POINTS

- The diagnostic medical interview should anchor around the patient's individual expression of their symptoms.
- The diagnostic medical interview should begin with open-ended questions and as it progresses use guided and hypothesis-driven questions intended to further the problem representation.
- Early learners should use system 2 based mnemonics to obtain a full history of present illness and to create a comprehensive differential diagnosis.
- Clinicians should obtain specific information about symptoms and background information that have significant likelihood ratios which will help narrow the differential diagnosis.

INTRODUCTION

Conversations between clinicians and patients happen in the pursuit of many objectives including building trust, rapport, and eliciting the patient's goals and values.[1] Although there is some overlap among these conversations, this article focuses on using the medical interview for the purpose of obtaining a diagnosis. In this context, the patient's personal experience and concerns are paramount. To conduct a diagnostic medical interview, the skilled clinician must come prepared with an approach to obtain a standardized medical history while also remaining flexible, cognizant of the uniqueness of each patient's story. This article covers the process of the diagnostic medical interview, from eliciting the patient's chief concern and history of present illness through the generation of a differential diagnosis.

[a] Department of Medicine, University of Virginia, Charlottesville, VA, USA; [b] Department of Medicine, Boston University, Boston, MA, USA
* Corresponding author.
E-mail address: jd3nd@virginia.edu

Med Clin N Am 106 (2022) 601–614
https://doi.org/10.1016/j.mcna.2022.01.005
0025-7125/22/

DEFINITIONS

What is diagnostic reasoning? For the purpose of this article, diagnostic reasoning begins with hearing the patient's story and concludes with making a diagnosis.[2] The process of diagnostic reasoning evolves throughout the medical interview. As more information is gathered, a broad list of diagnoses is narrowed to fewer and fewer options. The process used to make a diagnosis depends on the experience of the clinician and the complexity of the patient's presentation. In general, experienced clinicians predominantly rely on system 1 thinking which is a rapid and unconscious method using pattern recognition, whereas less experienced clinicians rely more heavily on system 2 thinking (**Table 1**). System 2 is used by clinicians of all experience levels when the patient's presentation is more complex (**Fig. 1**).[3,4] Using system 2 thinking in these circumstances increases diagnostic accuracy.[5]

"Data gathering" traditionally includes eliciting the patient's history, performing the physical examination, and obtaining laboratory studies.[6] In the 1970s, ultrasound, computed tomography, and magnetic resonance imaging became additional diagnostic tools.[7] Another significant change in the data gathering process was the advent of the electronic medical record (EMR), also introduced in the 1970s and becoming more widespread in the 1980s and 1990s.[8,9] The EMR greatly altered the data gathering process[10] by making large quantities of previously unavailable data accessible to clinicians.[9]

An "illness script" is the mental grouping of knowledge about a particular disease or syndrome.[2] The script typically consists of important epidemiology, clinical findings, and pathophysiology of the disease. Illness scripts are specific to each clinician based on individual firsthand experience caring for unique patients with that disease and change over time as this experience enriches.

The "problem representation" is a mental construction of succinct summary of the most salient features of the clinical findings gathered up to that point in time. Problem representations are frequently converted into written or oral form as the "one liner."[2] It typically includes important risk factors such as the patient's age, pertinent past medical history, and the presenting symptoms that are thought to be most contributory to the working diagnosis. It is at this point that the patient's medical history and symptoms are converted from the patient's language into medical terminology (**Box 1**). The clinician uses the problem representation to create and/or refine a differential diagnosis by comparing the problem representation to illness scripts.

In medicine, a "positive likelihood ratio" is a ratio of the frequency of a clinical finding (e.g., symptom or sign) that is present in a patient with a certain disease (i.e., sensitivity, or a true positive) compared with a patient without the disease (1-specficity or a false positive).[11] A "negative likelihood ratio" is the opposite. They can be used to help a clinician determine if a disease is more or less likely based on the presence of (positive likelihood ratio) or absence of (negative likelihood ratio) a clinical feature.

Table 1 System 1 and 2 thinking[3]	
System	**Definition**
System 1	Rapid and unconscious method of thinking that uses pattern recognition.
System 2	Slower and deliberate method of thinking that uses lists or detailed frameworks.

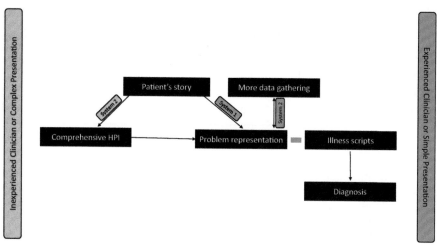

Fig. 1. Diagnostic medical interview based on experience.

APPROACH

Structure of the diagnostic medical interview

Typical structure of a comprehensive medical history

The diagnostic medical interview involves eliciting a comprehensive medical history (**Box 2**).

It is not entirely clear who originated the practice, but there has been a trend toward teaching learners to call the patient's primary reason for seeking care the "chief concern" rather than the "chief complaint."[12,13] The substitution of "concern" for "complaint" seems to be largely due to the negative connotation associated with complaining.[14] Particularly in the age of "open notes" when medical documentation is more widely accessible to our patients,[15] we need to reexamine and improve the language we use to describe our patients.

It is important to note the chief concern in the patient's own words. In a time of increasing automation of documentation in the EMR,[10] recording the chief concern at the top of the interview in the patient's specific language helps to mark the chief concern and the patient's voice as preeminent. The chief concern is the essence of why the patient sought care.

The diagnostic medical interview should begin with a patient-centered approach. This includes engaging the patient, introductions, and agenda setting.

Box 1

Example problem representation

Patient story: "Over the past few weeks I've been getting more and more short-winded. The other strange thing I've noticed is that my stools have gotten really dark, almost black in color... A few years ago, I went to the doctor because I was having this funny feeling in my chest. They told me I have atrial fibrillation. Since then, I've been taking medicine to keep me from having a stroke."

Problem representation: Mr Brown is a 67-year-old man with a history of atrial fibrillation on chronic anticoagulation who is presenting with subacute progressive dyspnea and melena.

> **Box 2**
> **Components of a comprehensive medical history**
>
> Chief concern
>
> History of present illness (HPI)
>
> Background health information
>
> Review of systems (ROS)

During this introduction, the clinician should take note of the environment to ensure the patient's comfort. For example, the clinician should consider adjusting lights and lowering down to eye level with the patient. A diagnostic medical interview consists of three phases to obtain a comprehensive medical history: open-ended elicitation, guided elicitation, and hypothesis-driven elicitation. Most of the interview is spent in the open-ended elicitation section with the guided and hypothesis-driven elicitation techniques used to fill in gaps and to gather more specific information that will inform the differential diagnosis. These phases are not linear, but rather, the interview moves back and forth between them as the problem representation becomes clearer and additional hypotheses are triggered by this information (**Fig. 2**).

Three phases of the diagnostic medical interview

Open-ended elicitation
"Just listen to the patient. He is telling you the diagnosis."

Sir William Osler.[16,17]

Open-ended interviewing[18] is a style that invites the patient to tell their story in their own words.[19] Eliciting the chief concern and history of present illness (HPI) is usually the bulk of the diagnostic medical interview. The clinician should begin the interview with an open-ended question such as "Please tell me, what brings you in today?" This approach will generally lead to the disclosure of more medical information than closed questions. As the patient shares their story, the clinician should use nonverbal and paralinguistic methods to encourage the telling of the story (nodding, affirming facial expressions, eye contact, and so forth).[18]

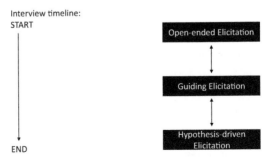

Fig. 2. Three nonlinear phases of the diagnostic medical interview.

Box 3		
Example of how question structure can introduce bias		
Opening line from clinician	How the patient begins their story	Focus of initial differential diagnosis
"I heard you were having chest pain."	"Yeah it started a few weeks ago..."	Cardiovascular system
"Please tell me what brought you in."	"I started having this chest tightness a few weeks ago."	Cardiovascular and respiratory systems

Even if you have already heard a version of the patient's presentation from another member of the care team, you should avoid asking questions that inappropriately narrow the focus of the interview as shown in the example later in the discussion (**Box 3**).[20] Such an approach may introduce bias.

An interview that starts off with a focus that is narrower than the patient's chief concern is at the very least less efficient and at worst could contribute to a diagnostic error.

Ideally, the patient finishes expressing themselves before an interruption to avoid the risk that valuable information will never be communicated from the patient to the clinician and to establish rapport. When studied, only about 25% of patients finished their response to the initial question posed in a medical interview and they were interrupted by a clinician after an average of 18 seconds.[21,22]

The use of guided elicitation to complete the history of present illness

Typically, after the patient provides their story, there are still some key elements not yet elicited that can inform the differential diagnosis. Guided questions give more direction to the patient's storytelling than the initial open-ended questions but still allow for the patient to use their own words to share their story.

The clinician can often begin the process of obtaining additional key information by considering what is missing from their understanding of the HPI and asking up to five additional guided questions, as pertinent (**Table 2**).

Especially for early learners, the use of mnemonics can also be helpful in identifying information that is missing from the HPI (**Tables 3** and **4**).[21]

A particular focus on the timeline and tempo (e.g., worsening) of symptoms is crucial as these features have a significant impact on establishing and ranking the differential diagnosis (**Box 4**).[12,14]

Table 2	
Guided questions: using the 4 Ws and 1 H for obtaining key features of the HPI	
What?	*What* were you doing when it started?
When?	*When* did it start?
Where?	*Where* were you?
Why?	*Why* do you think it happened?
How?	*How* did it start (sudden or gradual)?

Abbreviation: HPI; History of present illness

Table 3	
Using OP²QR²ST-A to identify additional key features of the HPI	
O	Onset
P²	Provocation/palliation
Q	Quality
R²	Region/radiation
S	Severity
T	Timing
A	Associated symptoms

Abbreviation: HPI; History of present illness

Hypothesis-driven elicitation

In the hypothesis-driven portion of the interview, the clinician asks targeted questions with a specific diagnosis in mind to gain information that will help them reorder, expand, or shrink their differential diagnosis. Even during this part of the interview, it is important to word questions thoughtfully to try and elicit the most accurate and comprehensive medical information. Asking questions that are very specific or encouraging the patient to answer in a specific way may lead to anchoring or premature closure biases which can lead to misdiagnosis (**Table 5**).[23,24]

For early learners, particularly if they have little experience with the patient's primary symptoms, it is important to consider a comprehensive list of possible diagnoses. The utilization of mnemonics can assist with this (**Table 6**) as well as frameworks (methods of organizing information) provided in online databases or texts such as Diagnosaurus, UpToDate, AccessMedicine, DynaMed, Frameworks for Internal Medicine, and The Clinical Problem Solvers.

More experienced learners will likely use, whether formally or informally, less comprehensive schemas when creating a differential diagnosis such as anatomic, "common things being common," and "can't miss" frameworks (**Fig. 3**).

While most experienced learners do a lot of the mental work of generating a differential diagnosis in their minds, it is often helpful for early learners to write their differential diagnosis. This can also help prompt the learner to ask hypothesis-driven

Table 4	
Using FARCOLDERS to identify additional key features of the HPI	
F	Frequency
A	Associated symptoms
R	Radiation
C	Character
O	Onset
L	Location
D	Duration
E	Exacerbating factors
R	Relieving factors
S	Severity

Abbreviation: HPI; History of present illness

Box 4			
Effect of timeline of symptoms on differential diagnosis for dyspnea			
Symptom (duration)	Dyspnea (hours)	Dyspnea (days)	Dyspnea (years)
Likelihood of PE	PE +++	PE +	PE _
Likelihood of PNA	PNA +	PNA ++	PNA _
Likelihood of ILD	ILD _	ILD +	ILD ++
Key: PE = pulmonary embolism, PNA = bacterial pneumonia, ILD = Interstitial Lung Disease _ = likelihood approaches 0% + = low likelihood ++ = moderate likelihood +++ = high likelihood.			

questions targeted at identifying symptoms that are consistent with a particular diagnosis (**Box 5**).

In addition to developing general knowledge about the risk factors and key features of common diagnoses, it is important for clinicians to learn features of the HPI or past medical history that have likelihood ratios which will significantly alter the probability of a particular diagnosis so they can ensure that they ask about these features when a particular diagnosis is on the differential (**Box 6**).[11] The most well-known reference for this type of information is the Journal of American Medical Association's Rational Clinical Examination Series.[25]

In addition to gaining a clear picture of the primary presenting symptoms, it is also important to understand the interplay of these symptoms and the patient's emotions. Many symptoms have an inextricable link with emotions. For example, pain and dyspnea can be significantly impacted by fear and anxiety (**Box 7**). The link between stress and other negative emotions and disease is likely underrecognized. For example, Takotsubo cardiomyopathy is a disease in which strong emotional stress is often identified as the inciting cause of the cardiomyopathy.[30]

Some interview questions can expand the history of present illness and uncover misconceptions or fears that the patient holds

Consider asking the patient, "What do you think it is?" We are living in the age of "Dr. Google" and many patients will have looked up their symptoms online before seeking

Table 5		
Minimize the introduction of bias into the HPI even during the hypothesis-driven portion		
Less ideal	More ideal	Why?
"Have you noticed that your urine has been frothy?"	"Have you noticed any changes to your urine?"	Asking the more ideal question gives more significance to the description of "frothy" urine than the less ideal question.
"Do you take your medications as prescribed?"	"How often do you miss your medications?"	Asking the more ideal question normalizes the act of missing medication and may foster a more honest answer.

Abbreviation: HPI; History of present illness

Table 6 A Mnemonic to help clinicians create a broad differential diagnosis	
V	Vascular
I	Infection
N	Neoplasm
D	Drugs
I	Inflammatory/Idiopathic
C	Congenital
A	Autoimmune
T	Trauma
E	Endocrine/Metabolic

care. It can, therefore, be helpful to get a sense of what the patient has read previously to build on reliable information and correct any misconceptions. Further, ask the patient, "What are you most concerned about?"[26] Although not necessary for every encounter, asking the patient about their greatest concern can be helpful when the chief concern is one that often engenders fear (e.g., chest pain) or when a terminal diagnosis is high on the differential (**Table 7**).

Past medical and surgical histories, medications, allergies, family and social histories (background health information)

Information obtained in this section of the interview serves as background information to further inform the history of present illness. Background information assists the clinician in prioritizing the differential diagnosis or even generates new diagnoses that were not originally considered (**Table 8**). This information is generally most efficiently elicited via closed-ended questions.

REVIEW OF SYSTEMS

Traditionally placed at the end of the interview, the review of systems (ROS) is a structured way of trying to identify any symptoms that were missed during the HPI from

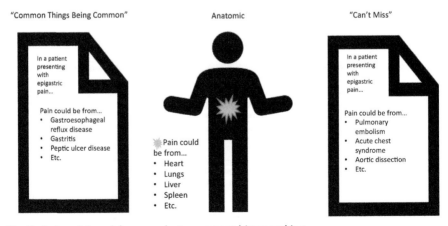

Fig. 3. System 2-based frameworks to augment history taking.

Box 5
Differential diagnosis for a patient presenting with fever and cough

Diagnosis	Risk factors, characteristic symptoms (+), uncharacteristic symptoms (-)
Viral bronchitis	Risk factors: sick contacts, history of recurrent bronchitis, immunocompromised state
	+: fever, rhinorrhea, pharyngitis, sputum production, cough
	-: dyspnea (unless history of asthma/chronic obstructive pulmonary disease)
Bacterial bronchitis	Risk factors: history of recurrent bronchitis, immunocompromised state
	+: fever, sputum production, cough
	-: dyspnea (uncommon unless mucus plugging or asthma/chronic obstructive pulmonary disease)
Pneumonia	Risk factors: immunocompromised state, history of recurrent pneumonia, history of chronic lung disease
	+: fever, *dyspnea*, sputum production, cough
	-: rhinorrhea, pharyngitis
Pulmonary embolism ("can't miss")	Risk factors: history of increased estrogen (e.g., pregnancy, use of exogenous estrogen), history of recent surgery, history of recent immobilization, history of malignancy, history of deep vein thrombosis or pulmonary embolism
	+: low-grade fever, *dyspnea*, cough, *unilateral leg edema, or pain*
	-: high-grade fever, rhinorrhea, pharyngitis, sputum production

---

overshadowing by the primary symptom(s). It can feel strange to ask such wide-ranging questions about symptoms that are unrelated to the patient's HPI at the end of the interview so it is important to keep the objective of the ROS in mind (**Table 9**).

CLOSING THE MEDICAL INTERVIEW

The clinician should ensure that the patient has no other questions, concerns, or issues to be addressed for example, by asking, "Is there anything else before we end?"[14]

Next, the clinician will move on to the physical examination and can make this transition by asking "Is it alright if I perform a physical examination now?".

CONSIDERATIONS
The electronic medical record

Before the advent of the EMR, the plethora of information now available would have been obtained by reviewing the much smaller paper chart or directly from the

---

Box 6
Examples of symptoms/risk factors with clinically significant likelihood ratios

Diagnosis	Symptom/risk factor (likelihood ratio)
Acute coronary syndrome[26]	Hx prior abnormal stress test (3.1), Hx of peripheral arterial disease (2.7), Radiation of pain to both arms (2.6)
Obstructive sleep apnea[27]	Nocturnal gasping/choking (3.3)
Severe upper gastrointestinal Bleed[28]	Melena (5.1–5.9)
Acute infection of a chronic wound[29]	Increase in pain (11–20)
Key: Hx = history.	

Box 7
Questions to help elicit emotional context

"What is this like for you?"

"How are you doing with this?"

"What does your cancer diagnosis mean to you and your support people?"

---

patient.[31] There are many benefits to the easy availability of medical data in the EMR including more efficient data gathering, particularly about the patient's past medical and surgical histories, medications, and allergies.[14] On the other hand, it can also lead to the creation of "chart lore."[10] Chart lore is incorrect or outdated health information that persists in the EMR and leads future clinicians to initially believe misinformation about the patient. Chart lore exists because note templates often automatically populate information about the past medical, surgical history, and so forth.[10] Clinicians will take the shortcut of referring to previously documented information about diagnoses rather than seeking out the primary source (or the primary source will not be accessible in the EMR). It is, therefore, imperative to double check the most important historical details that will impact the patient's care either from the patient themself or the primary source of data (e.g., pulmonary function test for substantiating a diagnosis of chronic obstructive pulmonary disease).

DISCUSSION

Patients are partners in the diagnostic process. Through the act of sharing their unique experience with symptoms, concerns, and questions, patients and their support partners work with the clinician to help make diagnoses.[32] This is a necessary shift to the traditional paradigm of diagnosis in medicine given the increased value placed on autonomy in medicine and the complexity of diagnosing and testing for medical conditions.[33]

A common trope clinicians make about the results of history elicitation that feels limited, incomplete, or confusing is to preface it with the phrase "the patient is a poor historian." Some clinicians take issue with this phrase for many reasons, not least of which is that it is an inaccurate use of the word "historian."[34] A historian[35] is one who writes about the past after studying primary sources.[36] In the case of medical history-elicitation, the patient is the primary, all-knowing source of their experience

---

Table 7
Deepen understanding of the patient's story

Chief concern	Answer to "what are you most concerned about?"
"I have a terrible headache."	"My father died from bleeding in his brain, could this be that?"
"I can't stop coughing."	"I know I need to stop smoking. This is probably lung cancer, isn't it?"

Table 8
Background health information

Past medical history	Includes all previously diagnosed conditions and approximate date of diagnosis.
Past surgical history	Includes all dates of prior surgeries and other procedures (e.g., colonoscopies).
Active outpatient medications	Includes name of drug, dose, route, and frequency. Should also include over-the-counter medications, herbals, vitamins, and supplements.
Allergies	Includes food and drug allergies and the reaction. Particular attention should be given to distinguish systemic reactions (e.g., anaphylaxis, dyspnea), rashes alone, or known adverse effects (e.g., cough from angiotensin-converting-enzyme inhibitors).
Family history	Includes health status of parents, siblings, and children. If pertinent, age and cause of death should be noted. Additional details should be obtained about conditions potentially related to the differential diagnosis (e.g., family history of breast and ovarian cancer in a woman presenting with a breast lump.)
Social history	Includes asking the patient about their living situation, social support, and independence in activities of daily living. Also should include questions about the use of alcohol, tobacco, and other drugs, occupation, and sexual history. This can also be an opportunity in the interview to learn more about the patient as a person by asking them what brings them joy and exploring the patient's values which may inform their choices about health care.

and the clinician is the historian. The main goal when using this phrase is to indicate to the listener that the history may not be reliable to obtain a diagnosis due to a real or perceived limitation in obtaining the full HPI. Therefore, instead of relying on this inaccurate and imprecise phrase, the clinician should more precisely characterize the limitations of the medical history. For example, the clinician can document that the history was affected by cognitive impairment, acute encephalopathy, language barrier despite the use of an interpreter, or low health literacy.

Table 9
The value of the background health information and the review of systems (ROS)

Chief concern (CC): "I haven't had a bowel movement in a week."	Identifying a history of appendectomy in past surgical history prompts the clinician to add obstruction from a transition point of the prior surgical site to their differential diagnosis.
CC: "I'm tired all the time."	Learning about a significant family history of early-onset colon cancer prompts the clinician to consider colorectal cancer as part of their differential diagnosis.
CC: "I'm getting winded going up the stairs."	Uncovering symptoms consistent with menorrhagia in the ROS prompts the clinician to add anemia to their differential diagnosis.

SUMMARY

This article covers the diagnostic medical interview which is targeted at obtaining a diagnosis for a patient's chief concern. The diagnostic medical interview has three main phases: open-ended elicitation, guided elicitation, and hypothesis-driven elicitation. The interview should always begin with open-ended elicitation which encourages the patient to share their story in their own words and move back and forth between guided and hypothesis-driven elicitation to complete the rest of the HPI. Using the patient's own words for the chief concern helps to maintain the patient experience at the forefront. The clinician should carefully consider the manner in which they ask the patient questions to decrease bias. The relationship between emotions and physical disease is likely underappreciated. Asking "what are you most concerned about" can help broaden the understanding of the patient's experience and concerns. Background health information and the ROS helps to expand or shrink the differential diagnosis. The advent of the EMR has enhanced the diagnostic medical interview process by increasing efficiency but also may lead to missed or delayed diagnosis due to inaccurate information. It is important to recognize that patients are our partners in the diagnostic process.

CLINICS CARE POINTS

- Use system 2 thinking when the patient's presentation does not closely match an illness script and therefore pattern recognition does not yield a diagnosis.
- Avoid interrupting the patient while they are telling the story of their symptoms and concerns.
- Refer to CC as "chief concern" rather than "chief complaint"
- Encourage early learners to use mnemonics such as the 4 W's and 1 H, OP^2QR^2ST-A, and FARCOLDERS to ask guided questions to fill in information about the HPI.
- Encourage early learners to use mnemonics like VINDICATE to formulate a comprehensive differential diagnosis.
- Frameworks such as anatomic, "common things being common," and "can't miss" can expand an initial differential diagnosis based on pattern recognition
- Knowledge of symptoms and risk factors of common diagnoses with clinically significant likelihood ratios improves diagnosis.
- Avoid the phrase "patient is a poor historian;" use more specific language about the limitation in history elicitation.
- Recognize that patients and their support partners are our partners in the diagnostic process.

DISCLOSURE

The authors have nothing to disclose.

REFERENCES

1. Sobel RJ. Eva's stories: recognizing the poverty of the medical case history. Acad Med 2000;75(1):85–9.
2. Bowen JL. Educational strategies to promote clinical diagnostic reasoning. N Engl J Med 2006;355(21):2217–25.
3. Croskerry P. A universal model of diagnostic reasoning. Acad Med 2009;84(8): 1022–8.

4. Marcum JA. An integrated model of clinical reasoning: dual-process theory of cognition and metacognition. J Eval Clin Pract 2012;18(5):954–61.
5. Hess BJ, Lipner RS, Thompson V, et al. Blink or think: can further reflection improve initial diagnostic impressions? Acad Med 2015;90(1):112–8.
6. Hampton JR, Harrison MJ, Mitchell JR, et al. Relative contributions of history-taking, physical examination, and laboratory investigation to diagnosis and management of medical outpatients. Br Med J 1975;2(5969):486–9.
7. Bradley WG. History of medical imaging. Proc Am Philos Soc 2008;152(3): 349–61.
8. Atherton J. Development of the electronic health record. AMA J Ethics 2011; 13(3):186–9.
9. Electronic health records: then, now, and in the future. Available at: https://www.ncbi.nlm.nih.gov/pmc/articles/PMC5171496/. Accessed September 29, 2021.
10. The impact of electronic health records on diagnosis. Available at: https://www.degruyter.com/document/doi/10.1515/dx-2017-0012/html. Accessed September 29, 2021.
11. Summerton N. The medical history as a diagnostic technology. Br J Gen Pract 2008;58(549):273–6.
12. Instructions for Write-ups » 3rd Year Medicine Clerkship » College of Medicine » University of Florida. Available at: https://clerkship.medicine.ufl.edu/clerkship-requirements/write-ups/instructions-for-write-ups/. Accessed September 30, 2021.
13. Siegel MD. The presentation series (The Chief Concern). Available at: https://medicine.yale.edu/news-article/the-presentation-series-the-chief-concern/. Accessed September 30, 2021.
14. Cooke M. Transparent charts and opening the problem list to patients. Available at: https://acpinternist.org/archives/2014/01/presidents.htm. Accessed September 30, 2021.
15. Federal Register: 21st century cures act: interoperability, information blocking, and the ONC Health IT certification program. Available at: https://www.federalregister.gov/documents/2020/05/01/2020-07419/21st-century-cures-act-interoperability-information-blocking-and-the-onc-health-it-certification. Accessed September 30, 2021.
16. Re: William Osler: a life in medicine. Available at: https://www.bmj.com/content/321/7268/1087.2/rr/760724. Accessed September 30, 2021.
17. Kravitz HL, Kravitz RL. Chapter 2. Subtleties of medical history taking. In: Henderson MC, Tierney LM, Smetana GW, editors. The Patient history: an evidence-based approach to differential diagnosis. 2nd edition. The McGraw-Hill Companies; 2012. Available at: accessmedicine.mhmedical.com/content.aspx?aid=56850014. Accessed October 1, 2021.
18. Dwamena FC, Fortin AH, Smith RC. Chapter 3. Patient-centered interviewing. In: Henderson MC, Tierney LM, Smetana GW, editors. The Patient history: an evidence-based approach to differential diagnosis. 2nd edition. The McGraw-Hill Companies; 2012. Available at: accessmedicine.mhmedical.com/content.aspx?aid=56850050. Accessed October 1, 2021.
19. Donnelly WJ. The language of medical case histories. Ann Intern Med 1997; 127(11):1045–8.
20. Lichstein PR. The medical interview. In: Walker HK, Hall WD, Hurst JW, editors. Clinical methods: the history, physical, and laboratory examinations. 3rd edition. Butterworths; 1990. Available at: http://www.ncbi.nlm.nih.gov/books/NBK349/. Accessed December 4, 2021.

21. Beckman HB, Frankel RM. The effect of physician behavior on the collection of data. Ann Intern Med 1984;101(5):692–6.

22. Fortin AH, Dwamena FC, Smith RC. Chapter 4. Clinician-centered interviewing. In: Henderson MC, Tierney LM, Smetana GW, editors. The patient history: an evidence-based approach to differential diagnosis. 2nd edition. The McGraw-Hill Companies; 2012. Available at: accessmedicine.mhmedical.com/content. aspx?aid=56850134. Accessed October 1, 2021.

23. Mamede S, van Gog T, van den Berge K, et al. Effect of availability bias and reflective reasoning on diagnostic accuracy among internal medicine residents. JAMA 2010;304(11):1198–203.

24. Kumar B, Kanna B, Kumar S. The pitfalls of premature closure: clinical decision-making in a case of aortic dissection. BMJ Case Rep 2011;2011. bcr0820114594.

25. The rational clinical examination. Available at: https://jamanetwork.com/collections/6257/the-rational-clinical-examination. Accessed September 30, 2021.

26. Fanaroff AC, Rymer JA, Goldstein SA, et al. Does this patient with chest pain have acute coronary syndrome?: the rational clinical examination systematic review. JAMA 2015;314(18):1955–65.

27. Myers KA, Mrkobrada M, Simel DL. Does this patient have obstructive sleep apnea?: the rational clinical examination systematic review. JAMA 2013;310(7):731–41.

28. Srygley FD, Gerardo CJ, Tran T, et al. Does this patient have a severe upper gastrointestinal bleed? JAMA 2012;307(10):1072–9.

29. Reddy M, Gill SS, Wu W, et al. Does this patient have an infection of a chronic wound? JAMA 2012;307(6):605–11.

30. Sharkey SW, Lesser JR, Maron BJ. Takotsubo (Stress) cardiomyopathy. Circulation 2011;124(18):e460–2.

31. Quinn M, Forman J, Harrod M, et al. Electronic health records, communication, and data sharing: challenges and opportunities for improving the diagnostic process. Diagn Berl Ger 2019;6(3):241–8.

32. Schiff GD. Diagnosis and diagnostic errors: time for a new paradigm. BMJ Qual Saf 2014;23(1):1–3.

33. Wijesekera TP, Sanders L, Windish DM. Collaboration of internal medicine physicians with patients and other health care providers in the diagnostic process. J Gen Intern Med 2019;34(7):1083–5.

34. Tiemstra J. The poor historian. Acad Med 2009;84(6):723.

35. Historians. Occupational outlook handbook: : U.S. bureau of labor statistics. Available at: https://www.bls.gov/ooh/life-physical-and-social-science/historians. htm. Accessed September 30, 2021.

36. Fisher JM. The poor historian': heart sink? Or time for a re-think? Age Ageing 2016;45(1):11–3.

Identifying and Managing Treatment Nonadherence

Jessica El Halabi, MD, MBI[a,1], William Minteer, MD[b,1],
Kasey R. Boehmer, PhD, MPH, NBC-HWC[c,*]

KEYWORDS

- Nonadherence • Multimorbidity • Partnering • Polypharmacy • Synchronization
- Health communication

KEY POINTS

- Medical treatment nonadherence is common, ubiquitous, and costs US $290 billion per year.
- Nonadherence often reflects a mismatch between patient and clinician priorities.
- Clinician interview and medication fill history, with or without integration with the electronic health record, are feasible ways to identify nonadherence.
- Evaluating nonadherence requires a nonjudgmental shared decision-making model to identify contributors to nonadherence and align treatment objectives with patient priorities.
- Treatment simplification is the most effective intervention for promoting adherence, whereas other interventions such as multicomponent pharmacy interventions, case management, consistent reminders and/or education, motivational interviewing, and reducing out-of-pocket expenses are also likely to meaningfully improve adherence.

INTRODUCTION

Chronic disease is an ongoing public health challenge. According to the National Health Interview Survey in 2018, more than half of adults in the United States have been diagnosed with at least one chronic condition; 25% of adults in the United States have one condition, and 27% have ≥2.[1] In the presence of multiple comorbidities, patients are often prescribed treatment for conditions individually, reflecting the single-disease nature of current clinical guidelines. It is estimated that managing a single condition such as chronic obstructive pulmonary disease (COPD) or diabetes according to guideline-concordant care can take patients 1 to 2 hours per day.[2] To the extent that additional conditions have cumulative or sometimes conflicting

[a] Internal Medicine Department, Cleveland Clinic, Cleveland, OH, USA; [b] Division of Community Internal Medicine, Mayo Clinic, Rochester, MN, USA; [c] Division of Health Care Delivery Research, Knowledge and Evaluation Research (KER) Unit, Mayo Clinic, Rochester, MN, USA
[1] Co-first authors.
* Corresponding author. 200 First Street Southwest, Rochester, MN 55905.
E-mail address: boehmer.kasey@mayo.edu
Twitter: @krboehmer (K.R.B.)

Med Clin N Am 106 (2022) 615–626
https://doi.org/10.1016/j.mcna.2022.02.003
0025-7125/22/© 2022 Elsevier Inc. All rights reserved.

medical.theclinics.com

tasks, this estimate increases. Often these enormous demands imposed by health care overwhelm patients and their caregivers, ultimately affecting treatment adherence.

Treatment adherence is defined by the World Health Organization (WHO) as "the extent to which a person's behavior – taking medication, following a diet, and/or executing lifestyle changes, corresponds with agreed recommendations from a health care provider," highlighting specifically that patients must be involved in and agree upon the plan of action.[3] Nonadherence occurs in instances where behaviors do not align with the agreed-upon treatment plan. More specifically, medication nonadherence can be subdivided into primary, when a patient receives a prescription but never fills the first dispensation, and secondary nonadherence, when a patient fills a prescription but does not take the medication as prescribed.[4] Primary nonadherence is estimated at 28%,[5] whereas secondary nonadherence rates for varying types of medication is estimated at 50%.[3] Other types of nonadherence, such as with dietary or exercise recommendations, are estimated to be at least 50%,[6] although in some circumstances this may be due to lack of counseling patients on appropriate diet and exercise regimens for their conditions.[6,7] Several studies show that nonadherence to chronic disease medications costs the US health care system more than $290 billion every year.[8] This led the WHO to consider it as a concern that requires urgent intervention.[3] Furthermore, treatment nonadherence is associated with increases in both morbidity and mortality across multiple conditions.[9,10] Beyond these important problems, the impact of nonadherence on patients' quality of life is substantial; about 40% of patients report that the burden of treatment as prescribed is unsustainable.[11]

The reasons that lead to medication nonadherence are multifactorial (**Fig. 1**). Beyond the cumulative effect of time spent managing multiple conditions, patients must normalize and cope with the work required to manage their illnesses. The work required includes sense-making, planning treatment tasks during everyday life, enrolling others to assist, enacting treatment, self-monitoring, and reflecting on the payoff in symptom improvement or long-term risk reduction after treatment implementation.[12,13] Fractured, uncoordinated care resulting from multiple subspecialists managing the same patient may exacerbate these issues. Importantly, lack of insurance coverage or the finances to afford prescribed medications represents a barrier to medication adherence.[14] Treatment fatigue, an intrinsic manifestation of the extrinsic burden of care, can lead to nonadherence and has been evaluated in chronic conditions including diabetes and chronic human immunodeficiency virus (HIV) infection. Patients may feel overwhelmed by how much time and effort is continuously needed to manage their chronic condition, ultimately leading to frustration and treatment nonadherence.[15,16]

To consider these issues practically, it is helpful to consider tangible examples of adhering to treatment. For example, a patient with COPD may be asked to use a nebulizer multiple times per day, or a patient with end-stage kidney disease is required to attend thrice-weekly dialysis appointments with sessions lasting 3 to 4 hours. In both cases, patients are required to understand the purpose of their treatments, alter their daily schedules, endure extended periods that can feel unproductive, and track symptoms after treatment. If these health care demands overwhelm a patient's capacity, defined as their available abilities and resources, it affects the self-management of their conditions. This in turn affects their health outcomes and quality of life.[17] Unrecognized workload-capacity imbalance and downstream consequences on adherence and health outcomes can also deteriorate the clinician-patient relationship, ultimately frustrating both well-meaning patient and clinician. This review outlines tools for the practicing clinician to identify, evaluate, and manage nonadherence across the spectrum of chronic disease.

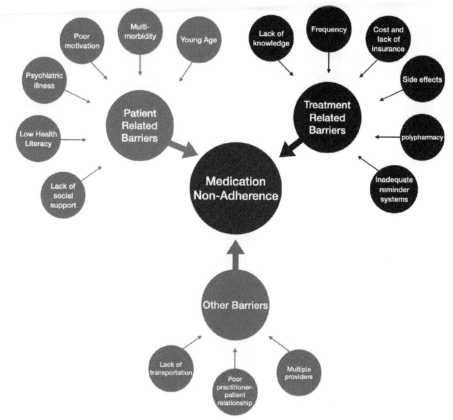

Fig. 1. Barriers that can lead to medication nonadherence.

EVALUATION

The first step toward reducing nonadherence is understanding the person's risk for nonadherence. Screening for a history of nonadherence risk factors (see **Fig. 1**) contributes to this risk assessment and optimizes medication reconciliation during each visit. Second, reviewing the electronic health record (EHR) is valuable in identifying insufficient refills, few visits, missed visits, or poor health outcomes, all of which are indicators of increased risk for nonadherence.[18]

Despite being an easily accessible tool, the EHR is not the ideal, sole source for identifying nonadherence.[19] For that reason, clinicians must rely on different ways to identify patients who are at risk for nonadherence. Several tools can be used by clinicians to measure and discuss patient workload, treatment burden, and capacity. These include Adherence Estimator,[20] ICAN Discussion Aid,[21] and various validated measures of treatment burden.[22–24] See **Box 1** for greater detail.

Beyond the use of conversation aids and validated questionnaires, **Table 1** lists sample questions for opening the conversation on treatment plan fit and evaluating risks for nonadherence.

APPLICATION

After identifying patients at risk for nonadherence, clinicians should strive to align a fitted care plan and incorporate the following interventions to support adherence. A fitted care plan results from the examination of guideline-driven pharmacologic and

---

Box 1
Tools to help measure and discuss patient workload, treatment burden, and capacity

- *The ICAN Discussion Aid.* A communication aid that can be used to assess patient capacity and treatment burden, as well as help tailor care plans to patients' lives.[21,54]

- *Adherence Estimator.* A 3-item screener (perceived concerns about medications, perceived need for medications, and perceived affordability of medications) for the likelihood for adherence to medications in individuals with chronic disease.[20]

- *Validated Measures of Treatment Burden.* These measures indicate the level of treatment burden experienced by a patient with multimorbidity.
  - *The Multimorbidity Treatment Burden Questionnaire (MTBQ)* is a 10-item measure derived from a British population that has been validated in the research setting and higher scores correlate with self-reported worse quality of life and higher disease burden.[22]
  - *The Patient Experience with Treatment and Self-Management (PETS)* is a measure with multiple variations (48-item,[23] 32-item,[55] 60-item[56]) validated in an American population; higher scores correlate with self-reported medication nonadherence, lower health literacy, and poorer health.[23]
  - *The Treatment Burden Questionnaire (TBQ)*[24] is a 15-item measure in which a Patient Acceptable Symptom State (PASS) which may be most useful in the clinical setting; patients with a score of about 59 on the measure are at risk for being overwhelmed by the current state of their medical care.[11]

---

nonpharmacologic treatments and the patients' unique situation, both biological and biographic. Upon examination, the identification of nonadherence to an existing treatment plan may signal that its value is unclear to the patient, it prioritizes health outcomes or quality of life factors that are unimportant to the patient, or that the work required to complete it is unsustainable given the patient's current capacity. Fitted care plans maximize patient-important health outcomes, quality of life, and sustainability over time.

Interventions to support adherence have been studied in common chronic diseases with a variety of interventions focusing on ameliorating patient, treatment, and health care system–related factors. It is difficult to draw firm conclusions from aggregated data of these interventions because of several factors, including heterogeneity of the diseases studied, participant characteristics, measures of adherence, classification and types of interventions performed, follow-up period, and measured outcomes. Regardless, improved medication adherence has been associated with improved blood pressure,[25–29] improved hemoglobin A1c,[30] and reduced emergency department visits and hospital admissions in older adults.[31] Systematic reviews of the literature have graded evidence ranging from moderate quality to very low quality for most of the interventions studied and caution is warranted regarding extrapolation of effect sizes to other populations and health care environments.[26,29,31–33]

Despite the limitations of the current literature, many of the interventions outlined below improve adherence and should be considered by the clinician after identifying barriers and eliciting patient-specific priorities. The etiologies of nonadherence are often multifactorial and as such, the interventions most often successful in the literature are composed of combinations of the interventions listed below.[26,27,31–34]

Patient-Physician Relationship and Eliciting Patient Perspective

Building a relationship with patients by eliciting and validating their perspective promotes adherence, trust, and improved patient satisfaction.[35] Often medical guidelines fail to invoke patient values, preferences, or capacity to adapt to change,[36] which is a missed opportunity for promoting adherence. Trusting relationships between patients

Table 1	
Patient-centered questions to assess treatment plan fit	
Questions	**Purpose**
What symptoms bother you the most? How might we address those within your treatment plan?	Connect treatment plan to patient-important symptom management.
What seems to be helping you right now with your symptoms?	Highlight and celebrate what is good; build upon what works.
What aspects of your life do you find the greatest joy in doing? • In what ways does your illness or treatment interfere with those activities? • In what ways does your current treatment plan support your continued participation in those activities?	Connect treatment plan back to the patient's life so the patient can understand what value potential treatment options may have. Identify targets for pharmacologic or nonpharmacologic interventions.
What aspects of your current medications do you find the most helpful? • What makes those helpful to you?	Assess what is working well; build on success.
What aspects of your current medications are most bothersome? • What makes them bothersome?	Assess what might need tailoring or support.
What aspects of your current treatment plan that are not medications do you find the most helpful (e.g., exercise, monitoring blood sugars, tracking food)? • What makes those helpful to you?	Assess what is working well; build on success.
What aspects are most bothersome? • What makes them bothersome?	Assess what might need tailoring or support.
Without any judgment, help me understand. How often do you take your currently prescribed medications? How often do you complete other activities to manage your health that have been recommended (e.g., diet, exercise, self-monitoring)?	Assess current adherence and potential need for tailoring or support.
On a scale of 1–10, how likely are you to be able to carry out the treatment plan we have decided together upon?	Assess feasibility of proposed treatment plan. Consider incorporating motivational interviewing.

and their doctors are associated with increased adherence even when the cost burdens of treatment are high.[14]

Medication Changes

Simplification of the medication regimen aims to reduce health care burden and is one of the most supported interventions in the literature to date. Discontinuing unnecessary medications, reducing the overall pill burden, prescribing single-pill combinations instead of individual medications, and changing medication frequency from multiple times a day to once a day are some of the interventions that most often demonstrate improvement in medication adherence.[26–29,31,33,37] Clinicians should aim to reduce medication complexity and elicit patient interest in single-pill combinations if insurance coverage allows and/or patients find the out-of-pocket costs acceptable.

Pharmacist-Led Interventions

Outside of the clinician visit, multicomponent pharmacist-led interventions improve medication adherence and patient education.[25–27,29,38,39] For example, synchronization of all medication refills to one date improves adherence and may improve Medicare Star Ratings score, which has reimbursement implications.[38] Dose administration aids including reminder packaging,[40] blister packaging or pill boxes,[33] may improve adherence, but often these interventions have been studied in conjunction with other pharmacy services, including education, motivational interviewing (MI), and medication counseling.[25,27,29,31] Shared practice agreements between clinicians and clinical pharmacists improve clinically meaningful endpoints including blood pressure.[25,26,29] Patients should be offered pharmacist consultation if this resource is available.

Patient Education

Reducing nonadherence with patient education alone has shown mixed results, with some averaged results showing only modest improvement.[33,41,42] Forms of patient education studied varied from printed or electronic education materials to in-person classes.[26,41,42] Structured education from many studies were conducted by nurses, pharmacists, or trained educators either in person or by phone.[26,41,42] Education may be most effective in reducing nonadherence with repeated sessions, serving also as a reminder.[26,30,41,43] Similarly, they may be more effective if implemented at the time of new diagnosis, instead of later in the disease course.[26] Although patient education alone has unclear benefits for medication adherence, combining education with other interventions such as case management improves adherence in the setting of cardiovascular disease, diabetes, and depression.[27] Case managers serve many roles in coordination, education, and referrals to programs and services that lower out-of-pocket costs.[44] Educational interventions, when combined with pharmacist-led interventions or case management may be more effective than educational interventions alone.[31]

Patient Monitoring, Reminders, and Feedback

Reminders or adherence feedback via letter, telephone, or electronic/text message have been studied in improving adherence. Most studies contacted patients with either scheduled reminders or triggered reminders after a patient did not refill a prescription. Similar to patient education, the results have been mixed with some demonstrating a small absolute benefit in adherence or clinical outcome, often of unclear clinical significance.[26,33,37] Personalized and interactive feedback may be more successful.[26,37] Studies implementing mobile devices have been difficult to compare, with low-quality evidence showing mixed results for improving blood pressure and cholesterol levels.[45] There is also no convincing evidence available at this time to suggest that providing adherence feedback to prescribers leads to large improvements in medication adherence or disease-specific outcomes.[46] Clinicians may still offer this intervention, if available and if patients are amenable, and tailor the form of the reminder to the patient's technological literacy.

Cognitive Behavioral Interventions

MI showed a small but statistically significant improvement in nonadherence in one systematic review.[47] MI cultivates intrinsic motivation and guides patients in creating individualized solutions to change behaviors. Most of the studies comprising the review focused on antiretroviral treatment for HIV. MI was conducted over varying lengths of time that were not correlated with adherence.[47] MI conducted by nurses and research assistants was associated with improved adherence compared with MI proctored by individuals with higher levels of education.[47] A different review grouping studies that investigate MI with other cognitive behavioral interventions showed mixed results on adherence, with many cognitive interventions co-occurring with other types of interventions, including adherence feedback.[26] In studies that reported positive results in reducing nonadherence, counseling was conducted over multiple sessions by a trained research assistant, counselor, nurse, pharmacist, or psychologist.[26,47]

Similarly, "Health and Wellness Coaching" is an emerging multicomponent intervention that uses MI among a variety of techniques to promote self-management. In 2016, a partnership between the National Board of Medical Examiners and the National Board for Health and Wellness Coaching established a national board certification process for Health and Wellness Coaching professionals.[48] Health and Wellness Coaching has been applied to patients with a variety of chronic diseases, showing reduction in perceived barriers to adherence or improvement in adherence in diabetes[49] and COPD.[50] Clinicians should incorporate MI when attempting to elicit patient preferences in formulating the treatment plan. They may also seek to enroll certified Health and Wellness Coaching professionals to support patients if available.

Health Care System and Financial Interventions

Reducing out-of-pocket costs for medications improves adherence according to multiple studies for cardiovascular and diabetes medications, but not inhaled corticosteroids per one systematic review.[27] Expansion of health care coverage, particularly among individuals who become eligible for and enroll in Medicare Part D, improves medication adherence.[51] Similarly, increases in copayments may increase medication nonadherence.[52] Alternative incentivization models that pay patients or primary care clinicians demonstrate mixed results. Although a conditional payment of $22 was associated with a modest improvement in monthly antipsychotic injections administered, studies that paid patients $8 per medication refill per month or used adherence-based daily lotteries were unsuccessful in meaningfully improving adherence.[26] When both physicians and patients were offered financial incentives, there was a small improvement in adherence and low-density lipoprotein level in one study.[26] Aside from conditional payments and regret lotteries, another financial incentive structure is a deposit contract.[53] In a deposit contract, patients offer up their own money and if successful will win that amount of money or more. If patients do not fulfill the objective, they lose their own money. One pooled analysis showed that conditional payments, regret lotteries, and deposit contracts can all serve as effective means of behavior change,[53] but as previously demonstrated, they can have variable effectiveness when broadly applied.[26] Change can include reprioritizing physician incentives[44] or eliminating barriers to accessing care, such as reducing long wait times or improving parking access.[34]

CONSIDERATIONS

There are several barriers or drawbacks to consider when enacting the above interventions to target improved adherence. These can be broadly categorized into patient and systemic. Patient-level challenges with adherence improving interventions include typically higher out-of-pocket costs for single-pill combinations, additional time burden for education, and inability to participate in deposit contract schemes if financial resources are limited. Systemic-level challenges include a lack of certain types of single-pill combinations for commonly coprescribed medications, lack of shared practice agreements

Table 2
Summary of interventions to support adherence

	Suggestions	Considerations
Medication Regimen Simplification	• Reducing pill burden, decreasing frequency • Single-pill combinations	• Counseling and coordination may increase visit time • Cost of newer medications
Pharmacy Interventions	• Medication therapy management • Synchronization of refills • Comanagement of chronic conditions	• Requires collaborative practice agreement • Not ubiquitous across systems
Patient Education	• Case management • Frequent, recurrent, educational sessions • Implement at diagnosis	• Single education intervention has unclear value
Monitoring, Feedback, and Reminders	• Personalized, interactive feedback • Increased medical touch-points	• Costs of staffing intervention
Cognitive Behavioral Interventions	• Motivational interviewing or health and wellness coaching • Can be implemented by clinicians or other trained members of the health care team	• Costs of training, staffing • Added visit burden to patients • Not ubiquitous across systems
Healthcare Policy Changes	• Reduce out-of-pocket costs • Reduce barriers to accessing care • Incentivize medication adherence	• Small patient incentives may not meaningfully improve adherence

between pharmacists and physicians in all health care environments, and additional staffing costs for education and coaching interventions to support patient adherence. Furthermore, federal funding policies dictate that pharmacists can be reimbursed for medication therapy management through Medicare Part D, but not through Medicare Part B.[25]

SUMMARY

In conclusion, nonadherence continues to be a challenge impacting clinical outcomes, quality of life, and health care costs. Being nonjudgmental and supporting patient engagement, in addition to using different tools to delineate patterns of nonadherence, is useful for identifying patients at risk. When nonadherence is identified, tailoring the care plan, simplifying the medication regimen, and incorporating multicomponent interventions that ameliorate patient, treatment, and health care system–related factors increase adherence and improve patient outcomes.

CLINICS CARE POINTS

- Recognize that enormous demands imposed by health care can overwhelm patients and ultimately affect their adherence to treatment plans

- When a patient has not adhered to the treatment plan, investigate why by exploring the numerous possible factors shown in **Fig. 1**
- Use nonjudgmental, supportive communication **(Table 2)** to tailor care plans and promote successful adherence
- To improve adherence, implement or improve interventions that incorporate medication simplification, pharmacist consultation, education with reminders, motivational interviewing, and/or reduced health care costs

DISCLOSURE

The authors have nothing to disclose. This research was supported by the Agency for Healthcare Research and Quality (AHRQ), grant T32HS026379, Patient-Centered Outcomes Research Institute (PCORI), grant K12HS026379, and the National Institutes of Health's National Center for Advancing Translational Sciences, grant KL2TR002492. Additional support for MN-LHS scholars is offered by the University of Minnesota Office of Academic Clinical Affairs and the Division of Health Policy and Management, University of Minnesota School of Public Health. The content is solely the responsibility of the authors and does not necessarily represent the official views of AHRQ, PCORI, or Minnesota Learning Health System Mentored Career Development Program (MN-LHS).

REFERENCES

1. Boersma P, Black LI, Ward BW. Peer reviewed: prevalence of multiple chronic conditions among US adults, 2018. Preventing Chronic Dis 2020;17.
2. Yen L, McRae IS, Jowsey T, et al. Health work by older people with chronic illness: how much time does it take? Chronic Illness 2013;9:268–82.
3. World Health Organization. Adherence to long-term therapies: evidence for action. World Health Organization; 2003. Available at: https://apps.who.int/iris/bitstream/handle/10665/42682/9241545992.pdf.
4. Raebel MA, Schmittdiel J, Karter AJ, et al. Standardizing terminology and definitions of medication adherence and persistence in research employing electronic databases. Med Care 2013;51:S11.
5. Fischer MA, Stedman MR, Lii J, et al. Primary medication non-adherence: analysis of 195,930 electronic prescriptions. J Gen Intern Med 2010;25:284–90.
6. Nelson KM, Reiber G, Boyko EJ, et al. Diet and exercise among adults with type 2 diabetes: findings from the third national health and nutrition examination survey (NHANES III). Diabetes Care 2002;25:1722–8.
7. Heymann AD, Gross R, Tabenkin H, et al. Factors associated with hypertensive patients' compliance with recommended lifestyle behaviors. Isr Med Assoc J 2011;13:553–7.
8. Lemstra M, Nwankwo C, Bird Y, et al. Primary nonadherence to chronic disease medications: a meta-analysis. Patient Prefer Adherence 2018;12:721–31.
9. Fitzgerald AA, Powers JD, Ho PM, et al. Impact of medication nonadherence on hospitalizations and mortality in heart failure. J Card Fail 2011;17:664–9.
10. Tohme F, Mor MK, Pena-Polanco J, et al. Predictors and outcomes of nonadherence in patients receiving maintenance hemodialysis. Int Urol Nephrol 2017;49:1471–9.

11. Tran V-T, Montori VM, Ravaud P. Is my patient overwhelmed?: determining thresholds for acceptable burden of treatment using data from the ComPaRe e-cohort. Elsevier: Mayo Clinic Proceedings; 2020. p. 504-512.

12. Gallacher K, May CR, Montori VM, et al. Understanding patients' experiences of treatment burden in chronic heart failure using normalization process theory. Ann Fam Med 2011;9(3):235–43.

13. May CR, Mair F, Finch T, et al. Development of a theory of implementation and integration: Normalization Process Theory. Implement Sci 2009;4:29.

14. Piette JD, Heisler M, Krein S, et al. The role of patient-physician trust in moderating medication nonadherence due to cost pressures. Arch Intern Med 2005; 165:1749–55.

15. Claborn KR, Meier E, Miller MB, et al. A systematic review of treatment fatigue among HIV-infected patients prescribed antiretroviral therapy. Psychol Health Med 2015;20:255–65.

16. Polonsky WH, Fisher L, Earles J, et al. Assessing psychosocial distress in diabetes: development of the diabetes distress scale. Diabetes Care 2005;28: 626–31.

17. Shippee ND, Shah ND, May CR, et al. Cumulative complexity: a functional, patient-centered model of patient complexity can improve research and practice. J Clin Epidemiol 2012;65:1041–51.

18. Kleinsinger F. The unmet challenge of medication nonadherence. Permanente J 2018;22.

19. Boehmer KR, Kyriacou M, Behnken E, et al. Patient capacity for self-care in the medical record of patients with chronic conditions: a mixed-methods retrospective study. BMC Fam Pract 2018;19:1–7.

20. McHorney CA. The Adherence Estimator: a brief, proximal screener for patient propensity to adhere to prescription medications for chronic disease. Curr Med Res Opin 2009;25:215–38.

21. Boehmer KR, Hargraves IG, Allen SV, et al. Meaningful conversations in living with and treating chronic conditions: development of the ICAN discussion aid. BMC Health Serv Res 2016;16:514.

22. Duncan P, Murphy M, Man M-S, et al. Development and validation of the multimorbidity treatment burden questionnaire (MTBQ). BMJ open 2018;8.

23. Eton DT, Yost KJ, Lai JS, et al. Development and validation of the Patient Experience with Treatment and Self-management (PETS): a patient-reported measure of treatment burden. Qual Life Res 2017;26(2):489–503.

24. Tran VT, Harrington M, Montori VM, et al. Adaptation and validation of the Treatment Burden Questionnaire (TBQ) in English using an internet platform. BMC Med 2014;12(1):1–9.

25. Marcum ZA, Jiang S, Bacci JL, et al. Pharmacist-led interventions to improve medication adherence in older adults: A meta-analysis. J Am Geriatr Soc 2021; 69(11):3301–11.

26. Kini V, Ho PM. Interventions to Improve Medication Adherence: A Review. JAMA 2018;320:2461–73.

27. Viswanathan M, Golin CE, Jones CD, et al. Interventions to improve adherence to self-administered medications for chronic diseases in the United States: a systematic review. Ann Intern Med 2012;157:785–95.

28. Parati G, Kjeldsen S, Coca A, et al. Adherence to Single-Pill Versus Free-Equivalent Combination Therapy in Hypertension: A Systematic Review and Meta-Analysis. Hypertension 2021;77:692–705.

29. Ryan R, Santesso N, Lowe D, et al. Interventions to improve safe and effective medicines use by consumers: an overview of systematic reviews. Cochrane Database Syst Rev 2014;CD007768.
30. Capoccia K, Odegard PS, Letassy N. Medication Adherence With Diabetes Medication: A Systematic Review of the Literature. Diabetes Educ 2016;42: 34–71.
31. Cross AJ, Elliott RA, Petrie K, et al. Interventions for improving medication-taking ability and adherence in older adults prescribed multiple medications. Cochrane Database Syst Rev 2020;5:CD012419.
32. Nieuwlaat R, Wilczynski N, Navarro T, et al. Interventions for enhancing medication adherence. Cochrane Database Syst Rev 2014;CD000011.
33. Anderson LJ, Nuckols TK, Coles C, et al. A systematic overview of systematic reviews evaluating medication adherence interventions. Am J Health Syst Pharm 2020;77:138–47.
34. Osterberg L, Blaschke T. Adherence to medication. N Engl J Med 2005;353: 487–97.
35. Haidet P, Paterniti DA. Building" a history rather than "taking" one: a perspective on information sharing during the medical interview. Arch Intern Med 2003;163: 1134–40.
36. Wyatt KD, Stuart LM, Brito JP, et al. Out of context: clinical practice guidelines and patients with multiple chronic conditions: a systematic review. Med Care 2014;52(Suppl 3):S92–100.
37. Kripalani S, Yao X, Haynes RB. Interventions to enhance medication adherence in chronic medical conditions: a systematic review. Arch Intern Med 2007;167: 540–50.
38. Nsiah I, Imeri H, Jones AC, et al. The impact of medication synchronization programs on medication adherence: A meta-analysis. J Am Pharm Assoc (2003) 2021;61:e202–11.
39. Lee JK, Grace KA, Taylor AJ. Effect of a pharmacy care program on medication adherence and persistence, blood pressure, and low-density lipoprotein cholesterol: a randomized controlled trial. JAMA 2006;296:2563–71.
40. Mahtani KR, Heneghan CJ, Glasziou PP, et al. Reminder packaging for improving adherence to self-administered long-term medications. Cochrane Database Syst Rev 2011;CD005025.
41. Ampofo AG, Khan E, Ibitoye MB. Understanding the role of educational interventions on medication adherence in hypertension: A systematic review and meta-analysis. Heart Lung 2020;49:537–47.
42. Cornelissen D, de Kunder S, Si L, et al. Interventions to improve adherence to anti-osteoporosis medications: an updated systematic review. Osteoporos Int 2020;31:1645–69.
43. Fitzpatrick C, Gillies C, Seidu S, et al. Effect of pragmatic versus explanatory interventions on medication adherence in people with cardiometabolic conditions: a systematic review and meta-analysis. BMJ Open 2020;10:e036575.
44. Cutler DM, Everett W. Thinking outside the pillbox–medication adherence as a priority for health care reform. N Engl J Med 2010;362:1553–5.
45. Palmer MJ, Machiyama K, Woodd S, et al. Mobile phone-based interventions for improving adherence to medication prescribed for the primary prevention of cardiovascular disease in adults. Cochrane Database Syst Rev 2021;3:CD012675.
46. Zaugg V, Korb-Savoldelli V, Durieux P, et al. Providing physicians with feedback on medication adherence for people with chronic diseases taking long-term medication. Cochrane Database Syst Rev 2018;1:CD012042.

47. Palacio A, Garay D, Langer B, et al. Motivational Interviewing Improves Medication Adherence: a Systematic Review and Meta-analysis. J Gen Intern Med 2016; 31:929–40.

48. Who We Are. 2021. Available at: https://nbhwc.org/about/. Accessed December 1, 2021.

49. Wolever RQ, Dreusicke M, Fikkan J, et al. Integrative health coaching for patients with type 2 diabetes: a randomized clinical trial. Diabetes Educ 2010;36:629–39.

50. Long H, Howells K, Peters S, et al. Does health coaching improve health-related quality of life and reduce hospital admissions in people with chronic obstructive pulmonary disease? A systematic review and meta-analysis. Br J Health Psychol 2019;24:515–46.

51. Zhang Y, Lave JR, Donohue JM, et al. The impact of Medicare Part D on medication adherence among older adults enrolled in Medicare-Advantage products. Med Care 2010;48:409–17.

52. Doshi JA, Zhu J, Lee BY, et al. Impact of a prescription copayment increase on lipid-lowering medication adherence in veterans. Circulation 2009;119:390–7.

53. Haff N, Patel MS, Lim R, et al. The role of behavioral economic incentive design and demographic characteristics in financial incentive-based approaches to changing health behaviors: a meta-analysis. Am J Health Promot 2015;29: 314–23.

54. Boehmer KR, Dobler CC, Thota A, et al. Changing conversations in primary care for patients living with chronic conditions: pilot and feasibility study of the ICAN Discussion Aid. BMJ Open 2019;9:e029105.

55. Eton DT, Linzer M, Boehm DH, et al. Deriving and validating a brief measure of treatment burden to assess person-centered healthcare quality in primary care: a multi-method study. BMC Fam Pract 2020;21:221.

56. Lee MK, St Sauver JL, Anderson RT, et al. Confirmatory Factor Analyses and Differential Item Functioning of the Patient Experience with Treatment and Self-Management (PETS vs. 2.0): A Measure of Treatment Burden. Patient Relat Outcome Meas 2020;11:249–63.

Motivating Behavioral Change

Erin M. Tooley, PhD[a],*, Anjani Kolahi, MD[b,1]

KEYWORDS

- Motivational interviewing • Health behavior change • Medication adherence
- Patient-provider communication

KEY POINTS

- Motivational interviewing (MI) can be useful in discussions between medical providers and patients.
- MI can help motivate patients to change behavior, reduce resistance and discord in a relationship, and ease burnout in providers.
- The goal of MI is to help patients talk themselves into change by developing discrepancy between the patients' current behavior and their goals, values, or ideals.

BACKGROUND

As the COVID-19 pandemic swept through the world, the discussion of the epidemic of chronic, preventable illnesses largely went silent. However, heart disease and cancer, largely preventable ailments, continued to be the leading causes of death in the United States.[1] As Americans, we may see more diagnoses of chronic illness related to disruptions in preventive health care and increased stress and risk behavior as a result of the pandemic. As most chronic illnesses are linked to the same short list of health behaviors—tobacco use, poor nutrition, lack of exercise, and problematic alcohol use—conversations about health behavior change between health providers and their patients continue to be vital.[2]

Unfortunately, patient education around health behavior change is often not enough to lead to lasting behavior change. Motivational interviewing (MI) in health care settings aims to help practitioners and their patients have more productive conversations around changing health behavior and medical adherence.[3] MI was developed by Bill Miller in the early 1980s through his work with patients with substance abuse. Clinical trials show benefits of MI in the management of a variety of medical conditions

[a] Department of Psychology & Public Health, Roger Williams University, Bristol, RI, USA;
[b] University of California, Irvine Medical Center, Family Medicine Department, Orange, CA, USA
[1] Present address: 101 The City Dr S, Orange, CA 92868.
* Corresponding author. Psychology Department, Roger Williams University, 1 Old Ferry Road, Bristol, RI 02809.
E-mail address: Etooley@rwu.edu

Med Clin N Am 106 (2022) 627–639
https://doi.org/10.1016/j.mcna.2022.01.006
0025-7125/22/© 2022 Elsevier Inc. All rights reserved.

including cardiovascular disease,[4] diabetes,[5] asthma,[6] as well as lifestyle changes promoting dietary change,[7] weight management,[8] and substance[9] and smoking cessation.[10] MI has also been useful in improving medication adherence[11] and adherence to other treatment regimens.[12]

DEFINITIONS

It can be tempting for medical providers to follow the "righting reflex" and tell patients exactly what and how to change. However, this "directing" style can paradoxically lead patients to resist change.[3] MI is defined as "a collaborative conversation style for strengthening a person's own motivation and commitment to change."[13] MI can help patients resolve ambivalence by promoting discussion about change and minimizing discussion against change.

Ambivalence

When physicians ask their patients to take new medications, undertake new treatments, or engage in lifestyle changes, they may be met with some resistance. Ambivalence is an expected and normal part of the process of considering change,[13] but can be uncomfortable. This discomfort can lead patients to ignore or suppress this conflict between change and the status quo or convince themselves that change is unwanted or too difficult, leading to further inaction. Ambivalent patients will often express language both for and against change; sometimes they will express more statements against rather than for it. However, MI helps the patient "talk themselves into change" by differentially evoking and reinforcing change talk.[13]

Change Talk

Change talk, or statements the patient makes that are in favor of change, can be divided into *preparatory* and *mobilizing* types.[13] Preparatory statements include statements about desiring a change, ability to make a change, reasons for changing, and need to change. Mobilizing statements, on the other hand, reflect more of a resolve to change the behavior; a movement toward behavior change. This includes statements describing a commitment to change, activation or preparation to change, and taking steps toward making a change. A common MI mnemonic for change talk is DARN-CAT or Desire, Ability, Reasons, Need, Commitment, Activation, and Taking Steps.[13] See **Table 1** for examples of each type of change talk. During a discussion, the more change talk used by the patient, the higher the likelihood of patient change down the road.[14] It is important for practitioners to use strategies to evoke change talk, to listen for it, and to reinforce it throughout an MI discussion.

Sustain Talk

Ambivalent patients often make statements that either favor maintaining the status quo or are specifically against change.[13] These are also described using the DARN-CAT mnemonic (desire to stay the same, an inability to change, reasons to stay the same, etc). Sustain talk is inversely related to patient change.[15]

APPROACH
The Four Processes of MI

Miller and Rollnick describe 4 processes that occur during an MI discussion: engaging, focusing, evoking, and planning.[13] These processes are not linear stages and they may vary in duration. During the course of MI, the conversation may flow from one phase to the next, phases may recur, and they may overlap. During the

Table 1
DARN-CAT—recognizing and eliciting change talk

Type of Change Talk		Definition	Questions	Examples
Preparatory Change Talk	D Desire	Expressing desire or "want" to change	"How do you feel about making this change?"	"I want to quit smoking." "I would like to exercise 3 times per week." "I wish I could take my meds more regularly."
	A Ability	Expressing capability to change	"How might you be able to do it?"	"I know I could do it if I wanted to." "I might be able to remember to take my meds if I set an alarm." "I can probably go to the gym twice per week."
	R Reasons	Providing arguments for change.	"What are some reasons you might want to make this change?"	"If I used protection, I would keep my partner safe." "If I take my meds, then I will feel better." "I would be healthier for my kids."
	N Need	Expressing "need" or obligation to change.	"How important is this change for you?"	"I ought to go to my appointments more regularly." "I really should be monitoring my blood sugar regularly." "I need to use my CPAP."
Mobilizing Change Talk	C Commitment	Expressing agreement or intention to change	"How ready are you to make this change?"	"I am going to get the flu vaccine this year." "I will go get the tests done." "I will take my meds every day."
	A Activation	Expressing movement in the direction of change.	"What might you do next?"	"I am ready to cut down my drinking." "I will call my primary care doctor to discuss it." "It's time for me to quit."
	T Taking Steps	Describing the actions they have already taken.	"What have you already done?"	"I joined a gym." "I put my pills in a pillbox and set an alarm." "I threw away all of my cigarettes."

engaging process, the goal is to establish a collaborative working relationship. *Focusing* involves developing a specific focus and direction. Rather than persuading, coercing, or telling the individual what and how to change, the *evoking* process involves eliciting the individual's motivations for change and how it should occur. Lastly, once an individual has expressed motivation and readiness to change, the *planning* process focuses on how and when the change will occur. Throughout the 4 processes, the practitioner focuses on 2 main goals: (1) establishing a "spirit of MI[16]" and (2) using the "method of MI.[13]"

The Spirit of MI

The spirit of MI refers to the practitioner's values and the way in which a clinician practices MI.[16] MI spirit is broken down into 4 key elements: partnership, acceptance, compassion, and evocation.[13] An effective MI practitioner both experiences these values and demonstrates them behaviorally with a patient. *Partnership* refers to the "active collaboration between experts," the patient being an expert on their own life and circumstances.[13] The clinician also creates an atmosphere of *acceptance* by minimizing judgment and accepting the patient where they are in the current moment. Practitioners work with *compassion* to promote the welfare of their patients and understand that their own conceptions of a patient's needs might not be fully accurate. Lastly, a focus on *evocation*, or pulling insight from the patient, is an important value within the spirit of MI. The clinician assumes that people have mostly what they need to make meaningful change, they just need help evoking their motivation and commitment to change.[13]

The Method of MI

Along with establishing a "spirit of MI," MI practitioners use a set of specific skills and strategies to direct discussion. The goal is to create opportunities for the patient to verbalize change talk and minimize opportunities for them to verbalize sustain talk. The practitioner actively reinforces instances of change talk and continues to elicit it throughout the encounter.[17] Open-ended questions, affirmations, reflections, and summaries (OARS) form the core interviewing skills used throughout an MI discussion. See **Table 2** for definitions and examples of each of these skills.

Although *open-ended questions* are an important way to learn about the patient, too many questions at once may make a patient feel as though they are being interrogated. Although some closed questions might be necessary for obtaining specific information, more evocative, open-ended questions are preferred.

Affirmations can increase patient engagement, reduce defensiveness, and increase openness to considering change. It is important that these statements be genuine (people are very good at recognizing flattery as a means toward an end) and that they are distinct from praise by focusing on the patient.[13]

Reflections, guesses at the meaning behind what a patient says,[18] can move the conversation to a new level or new direction. A simple reflection emphasizes that the provider is listening and hearing their words while a complex reflection shows a patient that their provider understands the meaning behind their words, but without overshooting. Reflections should be brief and purposeful; the MI clinician is choosing what to reflect and what to let pass by and uses reflections to highlight and draw out change talk. Miller & Rollnick recommend 2 to 3 reflections for every question asked.[13]

Summaries list related bits of information that the patient has brought up (eg, reasons for change), link information that the patient brought up to previous information, or transition to a new area by showing that the practitioner has understood the information thus far and is ready to move in a new direction.[13]

Table 2
OARS method of MI

Behavior	Description	Examples
Open-ended question	Invites an infinite set of responses.	"What do you do to manage your weight?" "How do you feel about the medications you are prescribed?" "How do you feel about your diagnosis?"
[a]Closed-ended questions	Elicits a yes-or-no answer or a limited number of responses.	"Do you exercise?" "What medications are you taking?" "How much do you currently weigh?"
Affirmations	Statements that recognize the patient's strengths, positive characteristics, or efforts.	"You've worked hard to bring down your blood pressure." "It's obvious that you take your health seriously."
Reflections	A guess at the meaning behind what a patient says.	
Simple reflection	Using the same words or paraphrasing what the patient said.	Patient Statement: "I'm just so sick of being in pain" Simple Reflection: "You don't like dealing with your pain"
Complex reflection	Adding meaning to what the patient has said by identifying an emotion behind the statement, highlighting something important, or emphasizing an outcome.	Complex Reflection: "You are at the end of your rope."
Summaries	Statements that pull together several different things the patient has said.	Pulling together all the pieces of change talk over the course of the conversation and listing them all together.

[a] Closed-ended questions are not a part of the OARS behaviors but are included to provide a comparison to open-ended questions.

Considerations

MI-adherent and nonadherent behaviors. Specific practitioner behaviors may also enhance or detract from the MI spirit of a patient interaction. These are referred to as MI-adherent (MIA) and MI-non-adherent (MINA) behaviors (Moyers TB, Manuel JK, Ernst D. (2014). Motivational Interviewing Treatment Integrity Coding Manual 4.1. Unpublished manual 2014. https://casaa.unm.edu/download/miti4_1.pdf). See **Table 3** for descriptions and examples of these behaviors. MIA statements often boost the collaborative and accepting nature of the relationship between practitioner and patient, whereas MINA behaviors undermine the MI spirit in an interaction and should be avoided.

Application

Along with the skills described earlier, the following application skills can be useful in applying MI to a patient encounter and *developing discrepancy* between the patient's current behavior and their goals, values, or ideals.

Table 3
Ml-adherent and Ml-non-adherent behaviors

Behavior	Definition	Ways to Demonstrate	Examples
MI-Adherent Behaviors			
Affirmations	Statements that recognize the patient's strengths, positive characteristics, or efforts	Genuine and patient-focused statements, distinct from praise	"You've worked hard to bring down your blood pressure" or "You're really on top of your blood sugar" or "It's clear you've done your research"
Seeking Collaboration	Attempts to share power or acknowledge the patient's expertise	1. Directly asking permission before giving information/advice 2. Indirectly asking permission before giving information/advice 3. Attempts to work collaboratively	"Would it be okay if we go over some information about how to take this medication?" "This is up to you, but you could take it after breakfast or after dinner" "Where would you like to go from here?" or "What do you think your best option is?"
Emphasizing Autonomy	Statements that put the control explicitly in the hands of the patient	1. Emphasizing that the decision is truly up to the patient 2. Emphasizing the patient's control	"You have the information, it is up to you what to do next" "How you go about quitting smoking is up to you, what you think will fit best with your lifestyle."
MI-Non-Adherent Behaviors			
Persuade	Explicit attempts to change the patient's mind or get them to change their behavior	1. Giving information (biased in a specific direction) without permission 2. Sharing concern without permission 3. Giving tips or solutions without permission	"You are unlikely to be able to drink moderately since you have a family history of alcoholism" "I'm worried you are going to develop an STI" "You should carry condoms with you at all times; that way you can't forget them."

| Confront | "Directly and unambiguously disagreeing, arguing, correcting, shaming, blaming, criticizing, labeling, warning, moralizing, ridiculing, or questioning the client's honesty" (Moyers TB, Manuel JK, Ernst D. (2014). Motivational Interviewing Treatment Integrity Coding Manual 4.1. Unpublished manual 2014. https://casaa.unm.edu/download/miti4_1.pdf) | Using a judgmental, negative, or disapproving tone to convey information or disagree. | "Well you wouldn't have an STI if you'd been practicing safe sex" or "There's no way that you've been taking your medication as prescribed with your blood pressure that high" or "If you continue to drink the way you do, you will end up with life threatening liver disease." |

Selecting a target behavior. As there are often many health behaviors that could be addressed with common health concerns, it is useful for the practitioner to think of themselves as a guide.[3] MI practitioners collaboratively discuss with the patient where they would like to focus first, and then bring in their ideas about behaviors to address. Unless the behaviors mostly coincide (eg, a diet high in salt AND saturated fat), it is advisable to focus on one behavioral target at a time.

Asking evocative questions. Probably the simplest way to evoke change talk is by asking open-ended questions.[13] An MI practitioner asks questions that elicit different types of change talk, such as DARN-CAT language (eg, see **Table 1**). One particularly useful question is called the ruler question. It can be used to assess and evoke change talk around the importance of the change, readiness to change, and confidence in the patient's ability to change. A clinician may ask the patient, "How important is changing your diet to you right now, on a scale from 0 (meaning not at all important) to 10 (meaning extremely important)?" A patient might give a moderate number such as a 3, which typically signals low importance. The provider would follow-up with "What makes you a 3, and not a 1?" This then evokes the reasons why changing their diet might be important, even if their initial rating is not very high. Clinicians may also query the possible extremes of the situation; ask patients to discuss the best possible outcomes if they do change their behavior and the worst possible outcomes if they sustain their current behavior. Similarly, practitioners might ask open-ended questions that help the patient remember what life was like before the problem arose (eg, before their diagnosis). They might also ask the patient to describe what their future might look like if they change, compared with what it might look like if they do not change. For example, "What might your life look like in 10 years if you continue taking your medication the way you do now?"

Values and goals clarification. MI practitioners may also ask patients about their personal values or goals for themselves. This provides rich opportunities to explore how the patient's current behavior either helps or hinders their work in life areas that are important to them. A very useful exercise is to ask the patient to describe their ideal life, a life in which they have reached their goals and are living in line with their values. Then the provider and patient can discuss how their current behavior fits with this image and what it would take to get there.

Informing and advising. Certainly, an important part of the medical visit is the provision of the practitioner's expertise and guidance. A medical visit may also include giving diagnostic information or assessment results. In MI, information and advice is given using the elicit-provide-elicit model[13]: a practitioner attempts to understand what the patient already knows, asks permission before giving advice or information, and then after giving that information, elicits the patient's thoughts or reactions. The provider recognizes that the patient has the right to refuse information and/or listen to the information and make their own decisions about how to proceed. Statements are carefully considered to avoid falling prey to the "righting reflex," which can evoke patient ambivalence.

Responding to sustain talk. Sustain talk is a normal part of the behavior change process and does not necessarily reflect "resistance" toward the practitioner.[13] Even if a practitioner is not attempting to elicit sustain talk, it is likely to come up with an ambivalent patient. However, sustain talk should not be ignored; this can feel invalidating to the patient. Sometimes just a simple reflection of the sustain talk validates the patient's experience and encourages them to reflect the other side of their ambivalence, the change talk. Practitioners might also use a double-sided reflection, a reflection that summarizes both the change talk on one side and the sustain talk on the other. For example, "While you don't love to exercise, you think it could give you more energy and reduce your pain" reflects first the sustain talk, and then the change talk at the end. A clinician might also choose to emphasize the patient's autonomy when sustain talk seems to outweigh the change talk. A statement affirming the patient's right to make their own decisions about their health can make the environment conducive to considering change.

Dealing with discord. In contrast to sustain talk, discord is less about the change process and more about the working relationship with the patient. Miller and Rollnick define discord as a disruption in the collaborative relationship which can be signaled by defensiveness, an oppositional stance, a patient interrupting, or just disengagement with the discussion.[13] It is important to recognize that the provider's approach can also lead to discord or make it worse. Sometimes, taking a "one size fits all approach," not validating the patient's experience, or attempting to problem solve when the patient is not ready, can lead to difficulties in the discussion. When a provider notices signs of discord, a validating reflection (eg, "it's understandable that you are so concerned") or emphasizing autonomy ("what you decide to do is really up to you") can go a long way. Validating the patient's concern and then gently moving away from a difficult topic can also be helpful. Lastly, if you suspect the discord is related to your approach, a genuine apology can ease the tension and help you move the conversation to a more productive place.

Making a change plan. The patient may give clues that they are ready to move into the planning process by verbalizing more change talk overall, particularly mobilizing change talk. A provider also might use the readiness ruler ("How ready are you to change on a scale from 1 to 10?") to ask how ready the patient is to change their behavior. However, if a provider moves into planning and finds that more sustain talk or discord appear, it may be beneficial to move back into the evoking phase. Once the patient is ready to begin planning, a practitioner helps to shape the discussion into a specific goal with a timeline and discusses the steps the patient will take to achieve that goal and potential obstacles that may arise. It is important to remember that this is still part of the MI discussion; a practitioner should still focus on enhancing the MI spirit of the conversation and use the OARS and the skills described earlier throughout the planning process.

CASE EXAMPLE: MEDICATION ADHERENCE

Medication adherence centers on the extent to which patients take their medications as prescribed and includes a wide range of behaviors such as filling prescriptions, following dosing instructions, and completing the course of therapy as prescribed. To demonstrate the spirit and method of MI, we present a brief case example of a primary care physician (Dr) in a clinic setting concerned that their 32-year-old patient (Pt) is not adhering to the HIV antiretroviral medication regimen. For brevity, the case example presents a patient with relatively low resistance to change.

1. Dr: I want to talk to you today about your HIV medication and how it's going. Would that be okay? [ask permission]
2. Pt: Sure, whatever.
3. Dr: I see that you've been prescribed Biktarvy. What's that like for you? [open question]

4. Pt: Yeah, the HIV doc changed me to that a few months ago. Well, I'm supposed to take it every day but I feel that taking it once a week is enough.
5. Dr: Tell me more about that. [open question]
6. Pt: Well I feel fine normally. But when I take the medicine I don't like how my stomach feels. Sometimes I get diarrhea, other times I spend the whole day nauseous.
7. Dr: Almost seems counterintuitive to be taking this medication. [Complex reflection]
8. Pt: Yea, I miss work or have to cancel plans too.
9. Dr: That sounds tough. Seems like you worry about the side effects of taking it. [validating complex reflection]
10. Pt: Yeah. Also, it's hard to take a medication every day.
11. Dr: You are being really honest about how you're taking your medications. [affirmation] What makes you take it once a week? [open question]

The physician's goal is to explore patient's understanding of the function of the medication and why they are showing some level of commitment to taking it. Avoid the temptation here for the "righting reflex" to fill in potential knowledge gaps about creating HIV resistance by not taking a medication daily and/or correcting misinformation about the HIV disease process.

12. Pr: I don't know. Just in case it will help.
13. Dr: Part of you thinks this medication might be beneficial for your HIV. [complex reflection] What does having HIV mean to you? [open question]
14. Pt: Well, it's a scary word but I feel fine so I don't think of it much.
15. Dr: You feel well so you don't have to think about it. [simple reflection] If we could fast forward 5 years, what do you imagine your life will be like with HIV? Best case scenario? [looking forward]
16. Pt: I don't know. Stay the way it is.
17. Dr: Stay the way it is, that would be the best for you. [simple reflection] And worst case scenario? [open question]
18. Pt: My levels are up. Or I'm dead, like in the movies.
19. Dr: Things could get worse. [simple reflection] What would it feel like, for you, if your levels started to rise? [open question]
20. Pt: That would be scary.
21. Dr: That would be scary, you want to stay healthy. [complex reflection]
22. Pt: Ya. I don't want to lose weight or get weak or sick. Or die.
23. Dr: You like your life the way it is now. [complex reflection] What do you think you could do to improve your chances of the best case scenario happening? What's realistic for you? [open question]
24. Pt: I could take the medicine more, find an alarm or something to remember better. But I also hate these side effects.
25. Dr: Part of this is managing the side effects of your medication but you could see yourself fitting in taking it daily into your schedule. [double-sided reflection] What is your understanding of how or why you take this medication? [eliciting what the patient knows]
26. Pt: I'm supposed to take it every day so the virus stays "quiet."
27. Dr: That's a good way to put it. [affirm] Is it okay to add on to that? (patient nods assent) Your goal is to maintain this undetectable level where the virus is not making you sick. So part of the reason you want to take it every day is so that it keeps the virus "quiet". Where do you see yourself going with that? [elicit-provide-elicit]
28. Pt: I don't know. It would be really upsetting to see my HIV numbers go up.

29. Dr: It'd be scary, it would be very upsetting. It would probably lead to some changes in your life. [complex reflection]
30. Pt: Yeah, I think if my HIV numbers go up I'd probably have more meds I'd have to take. And it would be scary to have sex, worry about infecting someone.
31. Dr: You're worried you could give HIV to someone else. [simple reflection] You've mentioned you're toying with the idea of taking the pill every day because although there are some side effects, you see some possible benefits. On a scale of 1-10, with 1 being not at all likely and 10 being very likely, how ready are you to take it daily as prescribed? [readiness ruler question]
32. Pt: 5? 6?
33. Dr: Why not a 3 or 4?
34. Pt: Because I do like how my life is right now. And I don't want to let it get out of control. Maybe I need this med.
35. Dr: Your health is important to you and maybe this med is needed to help you stay healthy. [complex reflection] Where do you see yourself going with that? [open question]
36. Pt: I'm going to do better at taking it every day.

From here, the physician should further strengthen the patient's commitment to changing their medication use, and help the patient develop a change plan. The doctor may also decide to bring in additional resources such as those to address the drug's side effect profile if the patient is interested in hearing about this and/or discussion regarding different therapies. However, the overarching spirit of MI maintains that although the physician is the expert in the medication and available therapies, it is the patient who is the expert in how, when, what, and most importantly why to change.

This article is meant to be a general overview of how MI might be used in these kinds of discussions. Those interested in formal training can attend a training workshop. For more information on training events, visit motivationalinterviewing.org. Additional training and supervisory feedback after a training workshop leads to enhanced competence in MI when compared with a typical 2-day workshop.[19] Nonetheless, everyone starts somewhere. Even simply incorporating some of the aspects of MI spirit and method described earlier may lead to easier medical discussions with patients.

DISCUSSION

As a medical provider, it can be frustrating when it feels as though recommendations go unheeded, which may lead to the impulse to give more information or advice. However, when a patient is "resistant," further instruction or advisement can create a difficult dynamic between patient and provider. Often it is this dynamic that leads to provider burnout over time. MI allows the provider to "let go" of the responsibility of patient behavior change and rather, guide the patient to reach their health goals driven by their own motivation and values. The practitioner should also let go of immediate expectations and consider change as a process, not as a singular event. Many times, once the seed of change has been planted, it will continue to grow in the patient's mind and change will come with time.

SUMMARY

MI can be a useful addition to medical discussions between patients and providers. It helps motivate patient health behavior change and may also reduce burnout in medical providers.[20] The MI spirit of an encounter, or the partnership, acceptance, compassion, and evocation exhibited by the clinician, and the MI-specific strategies used, such as the OARS, MI-adherent behaviors, and strategies to develop discrepancy, can enhance the patient's motivation and confidence in their ability to change health and medical adherence behaviors. For a new practitioner in MI, the technical skills of the process may seem daunting. However, MI is about the spirit brought to the conversation, as much as the techniques used. Behavioral change has to be thought of as an ongoing process. Starting the discussion is the objective for the provider, not necessarily changing the behavior in a single encounter.

CLINICS CARE POINTS

- Remember that the "spirit of MI" involves collaboration between you and patient on health goals centered on patient's priorities value system. You are not the "expert" for what, how, nor why the change will be helpful; the patient is.

- Ask open-ended questions instead of "yes" or "no" questions.

- Avoid the "righting reflex" in directing patients on exactly what and how to change. Especially when time is limited, it can be more helpful to ask the patient *why* they would want to make a change and *how* they might do it rather than telling them that they should change.

- Practice reflective listening with empathy to help highlight the patient's thoughts so that the patient may then reflect and arrive at an idea for what or how to change.

- Genuine affirmations can be useful. Focus on specifics and patient's efforts rather than your evaluation of those efforts. For example, instead of saying "I am so proud of you", the provider might say "you've worked hard to bring down your blood pressure!"

- Summarize the discussion to help the patient identify a specific goal.

- When you hear change talk, reflect and amplify it for the patient to hear themselves as well.

- It is important to "roll with resistance" without judgment and provide a simple reflection of the resistance or emphasize the patient's choice to change ("it's up to you").

DISCLOSURE

The authors have nothing to disclose.

REFERENCES

1. Ahmad FB, Cisewski JA, Miniño A, et al. Provisional mortality data—United States, 2020. MMWR Morb Mortal Wkly Rep 2021;70(14):519–22. Available at: https://www.cdc.gov/mmwr/volumes/70/wr/mm7014e1.htm?s_cid=mm7014e1_w. Accessed June 15, 2021.
2. National Center for Chronic Disease Prevention and Health Promotion (NCCDPHP). About chronic diseases 2021. Available at: https://www.cdc.gov/chronicdisease/about/index.htm#risks. Accessed June 15, 2021.
3. Rollnick S, Miller WR, Butler CC. Motivational interviewing in healthcare: helping patients change behavior. New York: The Guilford Press; 2007.
4. Hardcastle SJ, Taylor AH, Bailey MP, et al. Effectiveness of a motivational interviewing intervention on weight loss, physical activity and cardiovascular disease risk factors: a randomised controlled trial with a 12-month post-intervention follow-up. Int J Behav Nutr Phys Act 2013;10(1):1–16.
5. Chlebowy DO, El-Mallakh P, Myers J, et al. Motivational interviewing to improve diabetes outcomes in African Americans adults with diabetes. West J Nurs Res 2015;37(5):566–80.

6. Schmaling KB, Blume AW, Afari N. A randomized controlled pilot study of motivational interviewing to change attitudes about adherence to medications for asthma. J Clin Psychol Med Settings 2001;8(3):167–72.

7. Flattum C, Draxten M, Horning M, et al. Story M. HOME Plus: program design and implementation of a family-focused, community-based intervention to promote the frequency and healthfulness of family meals, reduce children's sedentary behavior, and prevent obesity. Int J Behav Nutr Phys Act 2015;12(1):1–9.

8. Wong EM, Cheng MM. Effects of motivational interviewing to promote weight loss in obese children. J Clin Nurs 2013;22(17–18):2519–30.

9. Bertholet N, Meli S, Palfai TP, et al. Screening and brief intervention for lower-risk drug use in primary care: a pilot randomized trial. Drug Alcohol Depend 2020; 213:1–5.

10. Borrelli B, McQuaid EL, Tooley EM, et al. Motivating parents of kids with asthma to quit smoking: the effect of the teachable moment and increasing intervention intensity using a longitudinal randomized trial design. Addiction 2016;111(9): 1646–55.

11. Palacio A, Garay D, Langer B, et al. Motivational Interviewing improves medication adherence: A systematic review and meta-analysis. J Gen Intern Med 2016; 31(8):929–40.

12. Ok E, Kutlu Y. The effect of Motivational Interviewing on adherence to treatment and quality of life in chronic hemodialysis patients: A randomized controlled trial. Clin Nurs Res 2021;30(3):322–33.

13. Miller WR, Rollnick S. Motivational interviewing: helping people change. 3rd edition. New York: The Guilford Press; 2013.

14. Moyers TB, Martin T, Houck JM, et al. From in-session behaviors to drinking outcomes: a causal chain for motivational interviewing. J Consult Clin Psychol 2009; 77(6):1113.

15. Miller WR, Benefield RG, Tonigan JS. Enhancing motivation for change in problem drinking: a controlled comparison of two therapist styles. J Consult Clin Psychol 1993;61(3):455–61.

16. Rollnick S, Miller WR. What is motivational interviewing? Behav Cogn Psychother 1995;23(4):325–34.

17. Miller WR, Moyers TB. Eight stages in learning motivational interviewing. J Teach Addict 2006;5(1):3–17.

18. Miller WR, Rollnick S. Motivational interviewing: preparing people for change. 2nd edition. New York: The Guilford Press; 2002.

19. Miller WR, Yahne CE, Moyers TB, et al. A randomized trial of methods to help clinicians learn motivational interviewing. J Consult Clin Psychol 2004;72(6):1050.

20. Pollak KI, Nagy P, Bigger J, et al. Effect of teaching motivational interviewing via communication coaching on clinician and patient satisfaction in primary care and pediatric obesity-focused offices. Patient Educ Couns 2016;99(2):300–3.

Delivering Bad News

David Harris, MD[a], Timothy Gilligan, MD[b],*

KEYWORDS

- Bad news • Empathy • Emotions • Hope • Communication • Health communication

KEY POINTS

- To deliver bad news effectively and empathically, we must learn to be comfortable to be in the presence of the strong emotions that often arise in response to such news.
- Preparing for and organizing bad news conversations, such as with an established framework, can make the challenge of these conversations easier.
- A key step is to assess the patient's understanding of their situation before giving new information so that the new information can be provided in a way that is informed by what the patient is expecting.
- Patients have varying needs and desires, and the balance of empathy and support versus information and planning should be tailored to the individual patient.

INTRODUCTION

Like many communication challenges, delivering bad news is a recurrent and predictable task in our lives. Yet, as with several other communication challenges, we often approach the task without a clearly conceptualized plan, without confidence in practiced skills, and with a sense of dread. The task is further complicated by various personality traits: a reluctance to disappoint people, a discomfort with strong emotions, a desire to be liked, a fear of being blamed or criticized, or a desire to avoid the sadness of contemplating adverse life events and suffering. Although giving bad news is sometimes cast as a health care challenge, the task arises throughout human relations with varying degrees of severity, and we learn some bad habits well before entering medical school. When breaking up with a romantic partner in high school or college, did we say "It's not you, it's me"? Did we say, "It's for the best. You'll be better off without me" or "Don't worry, you'll find someone new"? Did we try to have the conversation in such a way as to minimize the risk that the other person might cry or get upset, or did we just disappear on them so as to avoid having to tell them the news at all? When we did not want to go to a friend's social event, did we tell the truth or a white lie? When our

[a] Department of Palliative and Supportive Care, Cleveland Clinic Taussig Cancer Institute, 9500 Euclid Avenue, CA-53 Cleveland, OH 44195, USA; [b] Department of Hematology and Medical Oncology, Cleveland Clinic Taussig Cancer Institute, 9500 Euclid Avenue, CA-60, Cleveland, OH 44195 USA
* Corresponding author.
E-mail address: gilligt@ccf.org

Med Clin N Am 106 (2022) 641–651
https://doi.org/10.1016/j.mcna.2022.02.004
0025-7125/22/© 2022 Elsevier Inc. All rights reserved.

toddler dropped their ice cream cone on the ground, did we distract them with something else to avoid a meltdown? Many of us come into medical careers with practice in avoiding or minimizing the delivery of bad news. Learning to do it well requires not only learning new skills but also unlearning old habits.

These bad habits do not necessarily come from a bad place. Part of what makes giving bad news hard is our empathic response when we see the impact of the news. We tell a patient that they have a serious illness, and we feel the sadness we see them experiencing. If they start to cry, we may tell ourselves that we made them cry and thus that we hurt them. That feels bad. It is natural that we would want to avoid repeating the experience. We also may feel a responsibility for fixing all of our patients' problems, and giving bad news about something that we cannot fix can feel like failure. We may tell ourselves that the patient is not strong enough to withstand the truth about their situation, and that we thus have to modify reality into something more palatable to them. Or maybe we distract them by quickly changing the subject: "Your cancer has come back and there is a very exciting clinical trial of a new drug that I think may work for you." We cannot give bad news clearly, honestly, directly, and empathically until we become aware of these old habits and stop carrying them forward.

In this article, we discuss skills and best practices for giving bad news that help us avoid the pitfalls described earlier and thus do better for our patients and ourselves. One key practice that is indispensable is developing the ability to sit in the presence of strong emotion—be it sadness, despair, anger, or something else—without trying to shut it down, minimize it, or make it go away. Such emotions are a natural human response to hearing bad news. Part of our role is to prepare for strong patient emotion, to remain present, and to respond empathically rather than trying to persuade the patient to feel differently.

BACKGROUND: PATIENT PERSPECTIVE

When receiving bad news about their health, what do patients want and what do they find helpful? There is no simple answer to these questions. Different people have different needs that relate to where they are in the course of their disease and their life, their cultural norms, their personality, and other factors.[1] One of the fundamental challenges when delivering bad news is finding the right balance between empathy and emotional support, on the one hand, versus information and expert guidance, on the other hand. Patients want both but in different proportions.[2] Because the right balance differs from patient to patient and from encounter to encounter, adjusting our approach to the specific patient's needs on the day they are being seen is critical. Adapting to the individual patient requires learning who the patient is, what they want out of the encounter, what they know about their condition, what they want to know, and how they are coping with their situation. Starting off with curiosity, sincere interest, open-ended questions, and reflective listening provides a greater opportunity to learn the patient's perspective and prepares us to speak in a way that aligns with their specific individuality, circumstances, and needs.

APPROACH
Frameworks

When learning a new skill, it can be hard to know where to start. Learning to give bad news is no different. Published frameworks outline the steps of these conversations, which provide structure and can help us avoid missteps. We present 2 such frameworks in **Tables 1** and **2**.[3,4] Both highlight the same key points: preparation is helpful;

Table 1 **Spikes**	
Setting/Starting • Choosing a comfortable setting, include all important clinicians and family.	"I'd like to sit down and talk to you about how things are going. Are there people who you'd like to join us for that conversation?" "I'd like to start by having everyone here introduce themselves"
Perception • Understand what the patient has already heard	"What have you heard so far?"
Invitation • Ask the patient how much they want to know	"I'd like to talk about the biopsy results. How much information would be helpful to you?"
Knowledge • Share the news in a single sentence	"I'm afraid I have bad news. The biopsy shows that you have lung cancer"
Emotions • Respond to emotions before giving more information	"I can tell this isn't easy to hear"
Strategy and Summary • Talk about next steps and check for understanding	"Are you ready to hear about what we can do moving forward?"

ask what they know before you share what you know; give the big picture first, respond to emotion, and then share the details or next steps later. Although these frameworks highlight the important steps of delivering bad news, not all conversations will flow the same way and the frameworks should not be viewed as rigid structures so much as guideposts. Like other clinical guidelines, it is sometimes appropriate to depart from them, especially if a patient or family member is prompting you to do so. At the same time, skipping steps risks making our work harder, less effective, and more time-consuming. We recommend learning one of the models, practicing

Table 2 **Guide (from VITALtalk.org)**	
Get Ready • Know what the news means • Invite important people • Find a quiet place to sit down	
Understand • Understand what the patient has heard first, before adding information	"What have you heard so far?"
Inform • Use a one-sentence headline	"The scans show that the chemotherapy isn't working"
Deepen • Respond to emotions to deepen your connection with the patient	"I wish I had better news"
Equip • Share the next steps as you end • This is a good time for a summarizing statement, or using teach-back	"Tell me what you'll say to your spouse when you get home"

applying it, and then individualizing your approach so as to make it work for you and your personal style. With practice, it becomes easier to adapt the model to different patient scenarios. In the rest of the article, we expand on key skills that fit into these frameworks.

Seven key skills

Responding to emotions. When delivering bad news, we have multiple goals. We hope for the patient to understand and retain the information, to hold onto hope, and to feel that we appreciate the impact of the news on them and their life. Our recommendations are based on the following 3 premises:

- Intense emotions prevent patients from absorbing information
- Empathically supporting our patient's emotions helps them retain information and stay hopeful
- Emotions come in waves. Patients need us to shift fluidly between supporting them through emotions during a wave, and then providing information between waves.

A key to achieving these goals is noticing emotion and responding to it empathically. To respond empathically, we must carefully observe the other person, watching and listening for clues as to what they are feeling. It can help to imagine what it would be like to hear the bad news ourselves as long as we remember that different people react differently.

Empathic responses can be verbal and nonverbal. Empathic statements are commonly taught through acronyms like SAVE[5] or NURSE (**Box 1**).[6,7] The key ideas are to recognize and name the patient's emotion, acknowledge what they are going through, validate or normalize what they are feeling, and align ourselves with them as supportive partners in their care. Acknowledging and validating what they are feeling can help them feel seen and understood and hence less isolated. Alongside these are nonverbal signs of support, compassionate use of silence, and statements that reflect back to the patient what we have heard from them. In responding empathically, we meet patients where they are rather than try to persuade them to be somewhere else, and we allow them to determine when they are ready to proceed.

Responding to emotion is also key in ensuring that patients retain the information that we deliver. When humans are feeling, we are not thinking intense emotion keeps

Box 1		
SAVE and NURSE mnemonics for expressing empathy verbally		
S	Support	I will work with you to make sure you receive appropriate care.
A	Acknowledge	I know this news is difficult to hear.
V	Validate	Anyone would feel upset hearing this news.
E	Emotion naming	I can see that you are sad.
N	Name emotions	It sounds like you feel angry about this.
U	Express Understanding	I imagine I would feel angry if this were happening to me.
R	Express Respect for how the patient is responding or coping	I'm impressed with how hard you have worked to take care of yourself and follow the treatment plan.
S	Supportive statements	I'm on your side and want to do what I can to help you.
E	Explore emotions	"What are you most worried about?" "Tell me more about how you are feeling about ...."

patients from being able to fully listen to what we have to say. If we attempt to give information while they are in a heightened emotional state, they will leave with an incomplete or incorrect understanding of what we have said. Instead, we must wait until the emotion has passed to give information. To complicate things further, emotions that arise from bad news are variable. They can occur immediately after hearing the news, or they can be delayed. They can arise once, or they can arise in waves throughout an encounter. We must be able to recognize intense emotions as they occur in our patients and fluidly shift between providing emotional support and giving information based on their emotional state.

Premeeting planning. Numerous benefits ensue from taking time to plan and prepare for a bad news conversation. Such news often changes the trajectory of the life of the patient and their loved ones and mutual trust makes discussing such news less difficult. One way to quickly lose trust is to not know key pieces of information. Reviewing the chart carefully, speaking with relevant specialists or consultants, and confirming the findings of key tests, including how they compare to prior tests, are nonnegotiable steps before the bad news conversation.

Holding the conversation in an appropriate place at an appropriate time when the appropriate people can be present also makes it easier to have an effective meeting. Is there a quiet, private space with enough room for those who will be present? Does it need to be reserved in advance? Will the key people be present? These details matter.

Consider how you are going to share the bad news clearly in a single sentence. Can you strip it of medical jargon and put in plain language that anyone could understand? At a more existential level, it can help to consider what the "bad news" means to the patient and their loved ones. What does the news signify? How bad is it and how are they likely to respond if they understand this? How do you feel about the news and how are you going to respond if they have a strong response? Too often we enter important conversations in our work with a plan to just wing it and figure it out in the moment. We strongly advise against such an approach for bad news conversations. Planning and preparing can spare you grief and regret, and our patients deserve better.

Introductions and agenda setting. Bad news conversations with patients take place in many settings and various steps will thus be more or less relevant depending on the specific situation. When the meeting with the patient and their loved ones begins, share a brief summary of why the conversation is happening and obtain agreement to discuss serious medical issues. If you were not able to ascertain this previously, confirm that the essential people are present for such a conversation. If the patient wants a key person to be present who is not there, it is generally preferable to reschedule the conversation or, if acceptable, try to have the person join by phone.

If all the people in the room are not known to each other, introductions demonstrate a genuine interest in those present and build trust early. If multiple members of the health care team are present, each should explain their role in caring for the patient. Although it is tempting to get down to business, spending a few minutes creating a meaningful connection with the patient and family present is essential, especially if your relationship with the patient is only lightly developed, or if there is mistrust between the patient/family and the health care team. Building rapport should be done in whatever way feels authentic to the clinician. If nothing comes to mind, consider the following:

- Ask the patient and/or loved ones to share what has been hardest about the journey so far and/or what is most important to them at this point.

- If you have only recently met the patient, ask them what they would like for you to know about them as a person.
- If the patient is not present at the meeting (which can happen if they are encephalopathic or critically ill), ask their loved ones to share what the patient is like as a person or to share a favorite story about the patient.

These stories build trust. Patients want their doctors to know who they are as people. Bad news will be less emotionally harmful if they trust the person delivering it, and they are more likely to listen to recommendations made by a clinician when they feel like that clinician knows who they are.

After introductions, it is helpful to clearly set an agenda. First, share a brief summary of why the conversation is happening. This can be generic or specific (eg, "A lot has been going on with Mr. P's health, and I'm hoping we can talk about what it means." Or "I'd like to go over your biopsy results.") Then, ask what questions or topics they would like to cover. When asking for their agenda items, obtain a full list instead of pausing to answer specific questions as they arise. Once we have a full list, decide whether to answer some immediately, or whether it would make more sense to answer them near the end of the conversation. It is often most appropriate to delay these questions to the end of the meeting, as long as we say this explicitly to the patient.

Establish a baseline. After introductions and agenda setting, prioritize exploring the patient's and loved ones' understanding of the situation. Establishing a baseline is critical for determining how to begin and conduct the conversation. It also includes exploring the patient's emotional state, their health literacy, and the level of detail they find helpful. We may have learned some relevant information about these baselines from the topics and questions they brought up while collaboratively setting the agenda. Before providing information, it is key to know the patient's and loved ones' understanding and knowledge. They may have a very sophisticated or not even a very basic grasp of the illness. They may have beliefs about the patient's condition that are accurate or inaccurate. They may or may not be aware of key medical facts. They may have high or low health literacy. If we do not know where the specific patient lies on these continuums, there is no way to tailor the conversation to their needs.

A key question before giving bad news is thus some version of "What has your medical team told you about your condition?" or "Would you please share with me your understanding of what's going on?" or "What's your sense of how things are going medically?" depending on the specific scenario. The phrases "what do you know" or "what do you understand" risk being heard as testing the patient, and there can be benefits to choosing different words. If there are multiple, equally severe medical issues, ask general questions such as "What do you think are the biggest issues affecting your health?" It can be useful to pay particular attention to the language that patients use in their response and to mirror this going forward. Did the patient call it osteomyelitis, a bone infection, or sepsis? Did they use the word cancer, tumor, or mass? Clinicians often use these words interchangeably but introducing a new word to a patient might lead to confusion over whether this is a new diagnosis or related to a previous one.

Letting the patient talk first in this way yields multiple benefits. To the provider, it gives insight into the emotional and cognitive state of the patient and family. If they share feelings of anger or sadness, we can respond empathically until these emotions recede, and also prepare for intense emotions after delivering the bad news. Their description of the illness helps us to choose both what information is most important and relevant to share, and what language to use for sharing it. Furthermore, it is another way to give the patient and family control which builds trust and may lessen feelings of helplessness. Lastly, if the patient understands that things are not going well and is able to articulate it, this puts them in a more active, transmitting role rather than a more passive, receiving role.

Delivering the bad news. Before sharing the bad news, it can be helpful to give a "warning shot." Warning shots are signposts that notify the patient and family that what comes next is going to be unwelcome. This ensures that they give us their full attention and allows them to brace themselves emotionally. Examples of warning shots include:

- "I have some bad news"
- "Unfortunately..."
- "I'm sorry/sad to say..."
- "The results are not what we were hoping for."

After delivering the warning shot, give the bad news starting with a single sentence focused on the big picture. This is analogous to the headline of a newspaper article. Avoid jargon, euphemisms, and details early on and focus on the big, take-home message as it impacts the patient. Determine what additional details the patient wants to know later in the conversation if they do not ask immediately. After giving the big picture sentence, pause and allow for some silence so that the patient and loved ones can absorb and contemplate what they have heard. Take this time to assess how the patient is responding emotionally and wait to see what they say next. From this point on, decisions on how to balance giving empathy and support versus focusing on information and planning next steps will depend on cues from the patient. If the patient wants information, then they will likely get frustrated if we focus on providing empathy and support. If they are feeling strong emotion and overwhelmed, focusing on providing information and treatment planning rather than responding with empathy can feel cold and make them feel that we do not understand what they are going through.

It can be challenging to distill bad news into a single sentence. There are times when it feels impossible to do so. If it is proving difficult, it is likely there are multiple pieces of bad news, and that they should be delivered one at a time to ensure the patient understands and to prevent the patient from becoming overwhelmed emotionally. Some examples of how detail-oriented bad news can be changed into a headline are offered in **Table 3**.

It may also be helpful to consider our own emotional reactions to having to give someone bad news. The strong emotions we sometimes feel when delivering bad news can shape how we conduct our side of the conversation. For example, intellectualization is a common coping mechanism. This can lead to us giving more information than patients need or want while at the same time missing chances to support a patient's emotions. Other unhelpful coping mechanisms include false reassurance ("I'm sure things will work out"), minimization ("Things could be worse"), changing the subject, and abandonment. To prevent our own strong emotions from affecting how we deliver information, anticipate and address our emotions before we begin talking to the patient.

Giving further information
- Wait for the patient to prompt you before giving further information
- Avoid giving more information than they are ready to hear unless there is a clear imperative to do so

Table 3
Sample headlines for delivering bad news

Detail-oriented bad news (patient may be distracted or confused by the data and not understand the overall meaning)	"Big picture"-oriented bad news (preferred)
Unfortunately, the CT scan showed that there are new lesions in the liver and spine, as well as some growth in the mass in the right lung, although the left lung lesions are stable.	Unfortunately, the cancer is spreading
The biopsy came back as adenocarcinoma of the lung—that is a type of cancer. It is in your liver and bones too, so it is not curable but we can treat it. You are going to need chemotherapy and some radiation to the bone lesions to keep them from growing	I have some bad news. You have lung cancer. Later on: Unfortunately, this cancer is stage IV, which means that while treatment can slow it down, we cannot cure it
Your husband came into the hospital with confusion from liver failure, which had to do with his drinking. We have evaluated him for liver transplant but he is not a candidate because of his continued alcohol use.	I have some bad news...your husband has liver damage from his drinking. Later on Unfortunately, we cannot offer him a liver transplant
As you know, your mother came into the hospital with a COPD exacerbation and needed to be intubated. Unfortunately, at this point, we have not been able to get her off the vent and feel that we are going to need to do a tracheostomy.	I have some bad news...it's looking like your mom is going to need to be on a breathing machine for a much longer time than we had hoped, and perhaps indefinitely. Later on: Unfortunately, at this point, we need to consider doing a tracheostomy. What do you know about tracheostomies?

- Give the information in bite-sized pieces
- Use teach-back to confirm their understanding.

Although giving a headline is a helpful first step, there are likely other pieces of information that need to be shared. After receiving the bad news and processing their emotions, patients will typically signal when they are ready to receive more information by beginning to ask questions. If they are not asking questions but we think they are ready to hear more information, it is okay to ask them what more they want to know or if they are ready to hear more information. If they indicate that they do not want to hear more at that meeting, respect their limits unless there is an overriding reason that they need to know more at that moment.[8]

When providing additional information, keep in mind that patients retain more when we break the information down into smaller pieces, separated by questions that assess understanding (**Box 2**). To improve retention, include teach-back questions, either during the explanations or at the end. Avoid giving a mini-lecture on the patient's condition, as this results in very little retained knowledge.

Attending to hope. A sense of hope is essential for coping with adversity and yet some medical scenarios can feel hopeless. Depriving patients of hope can be harmful. In addition, denial can be a powerful and important coping mechanism for some patients as they struggle to maintain hope. Entire articles have been written on this subject. Here are a few best practices for sustaining hope. First, respect the limits patients

Box 2	
Providing information example	
Risky Approach	**Preferred Method**
"I'd like to talk to you about COPD. COPD is a chronic, progressive lung disease that is usually caused by smoking, or other inhalation exposures. Smoking causes changes in your airways that make it harder for air to exit the lungs when you exhale, which leads to buildup of carbon dioxide in the blood. We typically treat this with inhaled bronchodilators and steroids, which will get your lungs to open up. And it's very important to stop smoking so things don't get worse."	"I'd like to talk to you about COPD. What have you heard about COPD?" *"I know it's a lung problem, kind of like asthma?"* "That's right. It is a life-long disease of your lungs, and it's similar to asthma in that the flow of air in and out of your lungs is obstructed, and both diseases can make you feel short of breath. Have you heard anything about how COPD is treated?" "Is it with inhalers?" "Yes – treatment for COPD like yours is typically a steroid inhaler that's taken regularly, and an as-needed inhaler for when you feel short of breath. And it's very important to stop smoking so things don't get worse."

place on how much they want to know.[9] The questions they ask are a strong clue about what information they do and do not want. Second, there is evidence in other settings that empathy supports hope.[10] Third, discussing what they hope for can sometimes identify attainable outcomes—relief of symptoms, being present at a meaningful upcoming family event, being discharged home from the hospital—even if other hopes such as cure are not attainable.[11] Fourth, strongly aligning with and supporting the patient's needs can support a hope that they will receive attentive care during the course of their illness.

DISCUSSION

In addition to our own habits, the clinical environment and workflow poses barriers and challenges to giving bad news well. In both inpatient and outpatient settings, the pace of work is often brisk, leaving scarce time for delicate or complex conversations. In the inpatient setting, there may be frequent changes in the clinician in charge of the patient's care so that there is little time to develop a trusting relationship. Many hospitals have inpatient rooms with more than one patient per room, making privacy difficult. Medical culture can also get in the way: strong emotions are often viewed as unprofessional and clinicians are expected to be able to see the most horrible things happen to people without becoming emotional. Although our stiff upper lips can serve an important purpose, they can also make it challenging to transition into a softer, more human way of being with someone whose life has just been turned upside down by a medical event or diagnosis.

SUMMARY

Giving bad news is a relatively common event in health care. By taking it seriously as a procedure with defined best practices to learn and pitfalls to avoid, we can improve our performance and do better by our patients and ourselves. Key challenges include learning to recognize and respond empathically to the strong emotions that bad news often evokes, and learning to be comfortable staying present with people who are experiencing strong emotions without fleeing or trying to shut down or alter their emotional response. In addition, learning what the patient already knows and what they want to know allows us to tailor our approach to the individual. Similarly, watching and listening to the patient allows us to balance empathy and emotional support with providing information and planning next steps based on the specific patient's needs and desires. The bad news exists regardless of whether and how we give it. Giving it well cannot make the bad news better, but it can allow the patient to experience a caring and human connection at a difficult time, to feel that their experience is valued, to have their needs better met.

CLINICS CARE POINTS

When preparing to give bad news to patients and/or their loved ones:

- Review the chart, talk to relevant specialists as needed, consider the physical setting, and contemplate what the meaning of the bad news is to the patient.
- Decide in advance how you are going to share the bad news clearly in a single sentence.

When giving the bad news:

- Alert the patient to the fact that you want to discuss something serious.
- When applicable, assess what they know about their medical condition and what their expectations are before giving them new information.
- Deliver a warning shot that you have bad news to give and then give the news as a headline.
- Follow the headline with silence (let the patient respond first).
- Respond to emotion with empathy rather than with information.
- Balance empathy and support with providing information and planning next steps depending on the needs and desires of the patient and their loved ones.
- Respect the human need for hope, respect limits patients express on how much they want to know, and be careful not to let candor turn into harshness.

DISCLOSURE

The authors have nothing to disclose.

REFERENCES

1. Li J, Luo X, Cao Q, et al. Communication needs of cancer patients and/or care-givers: a critical literature review. J Oncol 2020;2020:7432849.
2. Back AL, Trinidad SB, Hopley EK, et al. What patients value when oncologists give news of cancer recurrence: commentary on specific moments in audio-recorded conversations. Oncologist 2011;16(3):342–50.
3. Baile WF, Buckman R, Lenzi R, et al. SPIKES-A six-step protocol for delivering bad news: application to the patient with cancer. Oncologist 2000;5(4):302–11.
4. VitalTalk. Serious News. Breaking bad news using the GUIDE tool 2019. Available at: https://www.vitaltalk.org/guides/serious-news/. Accessed December 5, 2021.
5. Windover AK, Boissy A, Rice TW, et al. The REDE model of healthcare communication: optimizing relationships as therapeutic agents. J Patient Exp 2014;1(1):8–13.
6. Pollak KI, Arnold RM, Jeffreys AS, et al. Oncologist communication about emotion during visits with patients with advanced cancer. J Clin Oncol 2007;25(36):5748–52.

7. Back AL, Arnold RM, Baile WF, et al. Approaching difficult communication tasks in oncology. CA Cancer J Clin 2005;55(3):164–77.

8. Curtis JR, Engelberg R, Young JP, et al. An approach to understanding the interaction of hope and desire for explicit prognostic information among individuals with severe chronic obstructive pulmonary disease or advanced cancer. J Palliat Med 2008;11(4):610–20.

9. Bergqvist J, Strang P. Breast cancer patients' preferences for truth versus hope are dynamic and change during late lines of palliative chemotherapy. J Pain Symptom Manage 2019;57(4):746–52.

10. Smith TJ, Dow LA, Virago E, et al. Giving honest information to patients with advanced cancer maintains hope. Oncology (Williston Park) 2010;24(6):521–5.

11. DeMartini J, Fenton JJ, Epstein R, et al. Patients' hopes for advanced cancer treatment. J Pain Symptom Manage 2019;57(1):57–63 e52.

Establishing Goals of Care

Alex Choi, MD[a,1,]*, Tara Sanft, MD[b,2]

KEYWORDS

- Communication • Goals of care • Family meeting • Advanced care planning
- Cultural competency

KEY POINTS

- Establishing goals of care (GOC) with a patient provides higher quality health care and avoids unnecessary medical interventions.
- A patient-led approach is an effective way to establish GOC.
- Various communication techniques (eg, ask-tell-ask, NURS, REMAP) exist to help physicians guide patients when establishing GOC.

INTRODUCTION

The 2001 Institute of Medicine report defines patient-centered care as "respectful of and responsive to individual patient preferences, needs, and values and ensuring that patient values guide all clinical decisions."[1] However, extensive gaps exist between patient and care team when establishing a patient's goals of care (GOC).[2–4] A 2019 intensive care unit multicenter cohort study found only 25% of discussions between physician and families of incapacitated patients involved patients' values and preferences. Among those that did, only 8.2% resulted in explicit treatment recommendations based on patients' values and preferences.[5] With little time and training on how to engage in GOC discussion, up to 53% of physicians do not know their patients' treatment preferences.[2,6] Even when patients explicitly express their GOC, 10% of clinicians will not prioritize patient preferences.[7] The COVID-19 pandemic has further exposed these gaps, particularly the provision of fragmented, single-disease–focused health care.[8,9]

Establishing a patient's GOC should involve the patient, physician, and whomever the patient requests, which could be family, friends, and/or other medical providers. One person may be the health care proxy, who is legally appointed by the patient to make medical decisions on behalf of the patient in case he/she cannot or wishes to defer.

[a] Yale Palliative Care Program, Yale New Haven Hospital, New Haven, CT, USA; [b] Survivorship Clinic, Yale New Haven Hospital, New Haven, CT, USA
[1] Present address 1: Yale University, Yale Palliative Care Program, PO Box 208028, New Haven, CT 06520
[2] Present address 2: 333 Cedar Street New Haven, CT 06510
* Corresponding author. Yale University, Yale Palliative Care Program, PO Box 208028, New Haven, CT 06520.
E-mail address: alex.choi@yale.edu
Twitter: @alexchoiMD (A.C.)

Med Clin N Am 106 (2022) 653–662
https://doi.org/10.1016/j.mcna.2022.01.007
0025-7125/22/© 2022 Elsevier Inc. All rights reserved.

APPROACH: HOW TO ESTABLISH GOALS OF CARE

Many methods have been developed to help establish GOC.[8,10–12] In this section, the authors provide essential skills that are present in many of these methods. The layout is designed to emulate an inpatient provider's in-person workflow but can be applied to other settings including outpatient and telehealth. Physicians should use patient-centered communication skills, instead of imposing a "one-size-fits-all" approach.[13–15]

Before Entering the Room

The physician's role in GOC discussion is to be able to provide medical knowledge of the disease including details of estimated prognosis, answer clinical questions, and make recommendations based on patient preferences. Therefore, it is crucial to be prepared before initiating a GOC discussion. This includes reviewing the patient's disease course, consultant recommendations, expected complications, and overall prognosis. For covering physicians or those who assume care from another provider, a thorough chart review or reaching out to the previous provider is recommended. The authors also highly recommend reaching out to any subspecialist or primary care physician involved in the patient's care, as they may have discussed GOC with the patient previously.

Establishing the perspective of various team members and their understanding of the reason for the GOC discussion should be performed before entering the room. Additional steps may include setting up language translation services if needed, discussing the planned steps of the conversation (ie, SPIKES mode[12]), and designating who will lead the conversation.

Before conducting the meeting, it is important to establish if the patient is open to discussing GOC, if they want anyone present, and if the timing is appropriate for all interested individuals. If the patient is not open to discuss, or if they request a specific person to be present, the GOC discussion should be scheduled when the patient is ready and all participants are present.

In the Room

The first step is to set the scene, which includes establishing a quiet, private environment, sitting down, and introducing every person in the room. Next, the physician should confirm that the purpose of the meeting is to review GOC and request patient permission to continue. After obtaining permission, the authors recommend asking the patient for a list of questions or concerns to make a shared agenda. One effective communication skill to achieve this is to ask, "What else?" The following is an example:

Physician: Before I share my perspective, I would like to understand what questions, concerns, or topics you are hoping to cover during this conversation.
Patient: I would like to talk about what treatment options I have at this point.
Physician: Yes, we can review that. What else?
Patient: I also want to know when I can be discharged?
Physician: Ok. What else?
Patient: Hmm…. That's all for now.
Physician: Ok, and I would like to go over the treatment course so far and discuss possible next steps. Out of these topics, should we start with a summary and discuss treatment options first?

In terms of delivering serious news, there are 2 approaches. One is to use the "warning shot," which consists of setting up the patient for hearing serious news.[12] A common phrase used is "I have some serious news to share with you. Is it ok for me to share?" A second approach is to use the "headline," which consists of forecasting the content of information to be shared. For example, "Your labs and imaging results came back. Unfortunately, they suggest your cancer has gotten worse." Between the 2 methods, research shows no difference in overall psychological distress or recall.[16]

After disclosing serious news, it is vital to listen, provide empathy, and follow the patient's lead. When the patient is ready, we can broach the next step. This is when clinicians should ask candid, open-ended questions about what is important to the patient. Sample questions are listed in **Box 1**.

Clinicians should follow the lead of the patient and keep dialogue open. An effective communication skill to use during this phase is ask-tell-ask.[17] The following is an example:

Physician (ask): Can you tell me about your cancer treatment?

Patient: I'm on my third-line treatment since March. My oncologist wanted to do a CT scan last week but here I am in the hospital instead.

Physician (tell, ask): I'm sure this is not what you planned. What was the plan after getting the CT scan?

Patient: To review it to see if the cancer responded.

Physician (tell, ask): I hope it shows good results. What is your expectation if the cancer still grows?

Patient: I'm not sure. We didn't discuss that.

Physician (tell, ask): I had the chance to talk with your oncologist earlier today. Is it ok if I discuss possible scenarios with you?

Patient: That would be great.

Considering the delicate nature of GOC discussions, using appropriate language is important. **Table 1** includes a list of risky phrases to consider avoiding and alternative phrases to use instead.

GOC discussions can be complicated for a variety of reasons. There are several published communication skills available to troubleshoot communication challenges in GOC discussions (**Table 2**).

At the end of the GOC discussion, the physician should provide a summary of the discussion and next steps. Next steps include what the physician will do, what the patient will do, and the next time communication will happen.

After Leaving the Room

GOC discussions can be emotional for everyone involved, including the physician. Debriefing with the care team to discuss what went well and what was challenging can often be helpful. The final step is to document the GOC discussion and speak with any stakeholders or family members. The summary and follow-up items should be clearly written, along with any specific goals the patient mentioned.

Box 1

Sample open-ended questions to ask during goals of care discussions

- Have you ever considered what you would want in a situation like this?
- What is most important to you at this time?
- What are some things you are hoping for?
- What does a good day look like for you?

Table 1
Examples of phrases to avoid in goals of care discussion and alternative suggestions

Phrases to Avoid	Alternative Suggestion
We can either do everything or nothing	We are shifting goals and will do everything we can to help meet these new priorities
I understand how you feel	I can only imagine how you feel
That decision was made by the physician before me so I do not know	I am not fully aware of the details of that event, but let me look into it and I will get back to you

Table 2
Examples of difficult scenarios and associated communication skills

GOC Scenario	Communication Skill	Example
Overwhelming emotion	NURS([17]; ACH[a])	Patient: (crying) *I don't know what to do. I don't know where to start.* Name: I can see how sad this makes you Understand: I think anyone in your situation would feel this way Respect: You have been through so much Support: No matter what, we will be with you every step of the way
Fixation on clinical fact or event that is clinically irrelevant to current situation or patient's values	REMAP[18]	Patient: *I can't believe this is happening. Things worked out just fine the last time I was admitted.* Reframe: I can only imagine how difficult it is to process this news. But we're in a different place now. Expect: I sense some disbelief. Can you tell me more? Map: With the current situation, what are your priorities? Align: If I may summarize, it seems not having pain and being with family are most important to you. Propose: After I leave this room, we will try to do A, B, and C to achieve your priorities. Does that make sense to you?
Unrealistic goals/hope	"I wish...I worry..." statement[8]	Patient: *I want to keep driving. It's the only way I get to spend time with my friends at the movies.* Physician: *I wish things were different too. I also worry that if you were to drive, you may harm yourself or others. Let's think of other ways to see your friends.*
	Holding hope[19]	Patient: *(terminally ill with incurable cancer) I am still hopeful for a cure.* Physician: I hear your hope for a cure. What else are you hoping for? Patient: *I hope to not be in pain.* Physician: It is ok to have multiple hopes. Let's focus on controlling the pain first.

[a] *Abbreviation*: ACH, Academy of Communication in Healthcare.

CONSIDERATIONS

Unique considerations exist for both patients and physicians when engaging in GOC discussions (**Table 3**).

Physician-Specific Factors

The role of the physician during GOC discussion is to provide accurate medical information about the patient's prognosis and answer any clinical questions. Challenges occur when prognosis is unclear, whether from lack of information, multiple comorbidities, or disagreement among medical providers.[20] Other barriers include lack of time and training in GOC discussion.[6]

A common concern by physicians is the fear that a GOC discussion may disrupt the physician–patient relationship. Studies show that patients prefer physicians who provide optimistic information over those who gave serious news.[21,22] Many of these studies are cross-sectional and/or analyze the patient's perception of all physicians instead of one with whom they have a developed rapport.[23] A more recent longitudinal, prospective study suggests prognostic discussions may increase the patient-physician therapeutic alliance.[23]

One precaution is the common practice of using code status as a gateway to GOC; this constricts the conversation to an impersonalized, procedure-focused checklist.[24] Also, an existing do-not-resuscitate order or advanced directive may be different from patients' wishes in up to 44% of cases.[25]

Patient-Specific Factors

Personal unreadiness to engage in GOC discussion is one of the biggest challenges for establishing GOC, and this may stem from fear of death, lack of knowledge, or being in "battle mode."[26] This challenge becomes more evident when the clinical situation warrants an urgent GOC discussion. In this situation, physicians should avoid rushing GOC discussions.

Lack of information is a well-recognized challenge for patients. With evermore treatment options and new diagnoses, it is difficult to expect patients to be fully informed without the guidance of a physician. During recent years, misinformation has become a growing challenge.[27] Most of the misinformation that patients bring to GOC discussions come from online sources, such as social media, blogs, and unreliable Internet sites. As a result, physicians must not only provide accurate medical information but also identify and correct misinformation.

Fragmented health care also contributes to patient confusion. For example, patients with multiple chronic conditions may have multiple "primary" physicians. A patient

Table 3 Challenges for physician and patient when establishing goals of care	
Patient challenges	Lack of patient readiness Lack of information/misinformation Language barriers Fragmented health care (lack of "big picture")
Physician challenges	Uncertain prognosis Lack of time Lack of training Provider disagreement Fear of disrupting physician–patient relationship

may ask for the "big picture," but a subspecialist may not feel comfortable presenting this information or may not know the answer. As a result, the patient can feel lost and "not heard."

Language difference is another challenge. Speaking in the patients' preferred language helps with end-of-life discussions.[28,29] English terms such as "palliative care" have no equivalent translation in many languages, placing additional difficulty in comprehending treatment options and transition of care.[30]

Cultural-Specific Factors

Among the 4 biomedical ethics principles—autonomy, beneficence, nonmaleficence, and justice—autonomy is heavily emphasized in the Western medical philosophy.[31] As a result, physicians in the United States feel morally obligated to disclose all information to the patient.[32] However, such expectations do not exist in many cultures.

It is imperative for physicians to be cognizant of cultural differences when establishing GOC.[33] For Asian and Pacific Islanders, where Buddhism, Confucianism, and Christianity exist, family members are expected to be key participants in medical decision-making for the elder.[34] Similar expectations are found in older Latine patients with breast cancer, regardless of level of acculturation.[35] Family members from such cultural backgrounds may share barriers such as fear of being criticized for seeking professional help for a dying loved one when the cultural norm is to keep health issues within the family.[36,37]

Within the Black community, mistrust toward the health care system is well recognized,[38] and this may lead to misconceptions about hospice services or perceptions that withholding treatment are equivalent to provision of inferior care.[38] In addition, accepting hospice services or withholding treatment may suggest giving up faith in God's power to heal.[39]

Cultural competency training can help clinicians conduct more culturally appropriate GOC discussions.[40] One effective approach is to apply Community-Based Participatory Research (CBPR).[41] CBPR involves forming ethnic-based focus groups, then integrating cultural recommendations into standard clinical guidelines.

One effective bedside communication technique is to say "tell me more."[17] The example of Mrs M is illustrative. Mrs M is a devout Muslim. During her hospitalization, nursing staff were concerned, as Mrs M kept getting out of bed unassisted even though she was placed on fall precaution care. Despite using translators, Mrs M continued to try to get out of bed without assistance. Meanwhile the patient's family was angry at the hospital because staff would not come to the bedside fast enough when the patient called. When asked to "tell me more," it turned out Mrs M needed to perform *Wudu*, a cleansing ritual, before each of her 5 daily prayers, and the only clean water was in the bathroom. As a solution, 5 individual clean water pots were set up at the bedside.

DISCUSSION

Physicians cite patient factors as the major barrier to achieving GOC, such as difficulty accepting a poor prognosis and disagreement among family members.[6] However, many of these challenges can be mitigated by the physician, who can provide information about prognosis and various end-of-life scenarios.

Advanced care planning (ACP) is different from GOC (**Box 2**). ACP is defined as "a process that supports adults at any age or stage of health in understanding and sharing their personal values, life goals, and preferences regarding future medical care. The goal of advance care planning is to help ensure that people receive medical

---

Box 2

Examples of questions asked during advanced care planning and goals of care discussions

- Advanced care planning (ACP)
  - "If you had low chance of neurologic recovery, would you want to have artificial nutrition?"
  - "If your heart were to stop for any reason, would you want us to perform CPR and provide electrical shocks to the heart?"
- GOC
  - "Unfortunately the labs and imaging show your cancer has progressed. Knowing this information, what is important to you right now?"
  - "This is your first admission to the intensive care unit. We consider this an opportunity to think about what your priorities are."

---

care that is consistent with their values, goals and preferences during serious and chronic illness."[42] They overlap in terms of laying out specific preferences that need to be made in the setting of a serious illness, for example, mechanical ventilation, vasopressors, and tube feeds. ACP is performed more often in an anticipatory manner with hypothesized situations. GOC is performed more often at the time of a significant medical event. In both cases, patients can make their treatment preferences into an official legal document or an advance directive. Examples of advance directives include Medical Orders for Life Sustaining Treatment and Physician Orders for Life-Sustaining Treatment.

SUMMARY

The need to establish clear GOC is well recognized. When establishing GOC, we recommend using a patient-led approach, with the physician using various communication techniques to guide the patient to express their GOC. Both patients and physicians require unique considerations. These considerations can be met by recognizing their existence, communicating with an open-minded approach, and exercising cultural competency.

CLINICS CARE POINTS

- Up to 53% of physicians do not know their patients' end-of-life treatment preferences. Goals of care discussions help elicit such patient values.
- Before entering the patient room to establish GOC, be well prepared to answer any clinical questions and review team member perspectives.
- In the room, use a patient-centered approach when establishing GOC, using communication techniques such as "what else," open-ended questions, and ask-tell-ask.
- Tools can be helpful to show empathy (NURS statements) and further the discussion of new priorities (REMAP).
- After GOC discussion, check your emotional safety and debrief if necessary before documenting the GOC discussion and speaking with key stakeholders.
- Be aware of ethnic/cultural norms and preferences when establishing GOC. Avoid using code status as a gateway to discuss GOC.

DISCLOSURE

The authors have nothing to disclose.

REFERENCES

1. Institute of Medicine. Crossing the quality Chasm: a new health system for the 21st Century. Washington (DC): National Academies Press; 2001. p. 3.
2. The SUPPORT Principal Investigators. A controlled trial to improve care for seriously ill hospitalized patients. The study to understand prognoses and preferences for outcomes and risks of treatments (SUPPORT). JAMA 1995;274(20): 1591–8 [Erratum appears in JAMA 1996; 24;275(16): 1232].
3. Last Acts. Means to a Better End: A Report on Dying in America Today. Wasington, DC: Last Acts; 2002.
4. Institute of Medicine. Dying in America: improving quality and honoring individual preferences near the end-of-life. Washington (DC): The National Academies Press; 2015.
5. Scheunemann LP, Ernecoff NC, Buddadhumaruk P, et al. Clinician-family communication about patients' values and preferences in intensive care units. JAMA Intern Med 2019;179:676–84.
6. You JJ, Downar J, Fowler RA, et al. Barriers to goals of care discussions with seriously ill hospitalized patients and their families: a multicenter survey of clinicians. JAMA Intern Med 2015;175:549–56.
7. Haliko S, Downs J, Mohan D, et al. Hospital-based physicians' intubation decisions and associated mental models when managing a critically and terminally ill older patient. Med Decis Making 2018;38:344–54.
8. Tinetti ME, Costello DM, Naik AD, et al. Outcome goals and health care preferences of older adults with multiple chronic conditions. JAMA Netw Open 2021; 4:e211271.
9. Curtis JR, Kross EK, Stapleton RD. The importance of addressing advance care planning and decisions about do-not-resuscitate orders during novel Coronavirus 2019 (COVID-19). JAMA 2020;323:1771–2.
10. Paladino J, Bernacki R, Neville BA, et al. Evaluating an intervention to improve communication between oncology clinicians and patients with life-limiting cancer: a cluster randomized clinical trial of the serious illness care program. JAMA Oncol 2019;5:801–9.
11. Arnold RM, Back AL, Barnato AE, et al. The Critical Care Communication project: improving fellows' communication skills. J Crit Care 2015;30:250–4.
12. Baile WF, Buckman R, Lenzi R, et al. SPIKES-A six-step protocol for delivering bad news: application to the patient with cancer. Oncologist 2000;5:302–11.
13. Petrillo LA, McMahan RD, Tang V, et al. Older adult and surrogate perspectives on serious, difficult, and important medical decisions. J Am Geriatr Soc 2018; 66:1515–23.
14. Periyakoil VS, Neri E, Kraemer H. Common items on a bucket list. J Palliat Med 2018;21:652–8.
15. Johnson SB, Butow PN, Bell ML, et al. A randomised controlled trial of an advance care planning intervention for patients with incurable cancer. Br J Cancer 2018;119:1182–90.
16. Porensky EK, Carpenter BD. Breaking bad news: effects of forecasting diagnosis and framing prognosis. Patient Educ Couns 2016;99:68–76.
17. Back AL, Arnold RM, Baile WF, et al. Approaching difficult communication tasks in oncology. CA Cancer J Clin 2005;55:164–77.
18. Childers JW, Back AL, Tulsky JA, et al. REMAP: a framework for goals of care conversations. J Oncol Pract 2017;13:e844–50.

19. Rosenberg A, Arnold RM, Schenker Y. Holding Hope for Patients With Serious Illness. JAMA 2021;326(13):1259–60.
20. Boyd CM, Wolff JL, Giovannetti E, et al. Health care task difficulty among older adults with multimorbidity. Med Care 2014;52:S118.
21. Tanco K, Rhondali W, Perez-Cruz P, et al. Patient perception of physician compassion after a more optimistic vs a less optimistic message: a randomized clinical trial. JAMA Oncol 2015;1:176–83.
22. Gordon EJ, Daugherty CK. 'Hitting you over the head': oncologists' disclosure of prognosis to advanced cancer patients. Bioethics 2003;17:142–68.
23. Fenton JJ, Duberstein PR, Kravitz RL, et al. Impact of prognostic discussions on the patient-physician relationship: Prospective Cohort Study. J Clin Oncol 2018; 36:225–30.
24. Becker C, Lecheler L, Hochstrasser S, et al. Association of communication interventions to discuss code status with patient decisions for do-not-resuscitate orders: a systematic review and meta-analysis. JAMA Netw open 2019;2:e195033–.
25. Mirarchi FL, Juhasz K, Cooney TE, et al. TRIAD XII: are patients aware of and agree with DNR or POLST orders in their medical records. J Patient Saf 2019; 15:230.
26. Niranjan SJ, Huang CS, Dionne-Odom JN, et al. Lay patient navigators' perspectives of barriers, facilitators and training needs in initiating advance care planning conversations with older patients with cancer. J Palliat Care 2018;33:70–8.
27. Wang Y, McKee M, Torbica A, et al. Systematic literature review on the spread of health-related misinformation on social media. Soc Sci Med 2019;240:112552.
28. Heyman JC, Gutheil IA. Older Latinos' attitudes toward and comfort with end-of-life planning. Health Soc Work 2010;35:17–26.
29. Perry E, Swartz J, Brown S, et al. Peer mentoring: a culturally sensitive approach to end-of-life planning for long-term dialysis patients. Am J Kidney Dis 2005;46: 111–9.
30. Kirby E, Lwin Z, Kenny K, Broom A, Birman H, Good P. It doesn't exist...": negotiating palliative care from a culturally and linguistically diverse patient and caregiver perspective. BMC Palliat Care 2018;17:1–10.
31. Blackhall LJ, Murphy ST, Frank G, et al. Ethnicity and attitudes toward patient autonomy. JAMA 1995;274:820–5.
32. Gordon DR. Tenacious assumptions in Western medicine, Biomedicine examined. Dordrecht: Springer; 1988. p. 19–56.
33. Periyakoil VS, Neri E, Kraemer H. Patient-Reported Barriers to High-Quality, End-of-Life Care: A Multiethnic, Multilingual, Mixed-Methods Study. J Palliat Med 2016;19:373–9.
34. Giger JN, Davidhizar R. The Giger and Davidhizar transcultural assessment model. J Transcult Nurs 2002;13:185–8 [discussion: 200-1].
35. Maly RC, Umezawa Y, Ratliff CT, et al. Racial/ethnic group differences in treatment decision-making and treatment received among older breast carcinoma patients. Cancer 2006;106:957–65.
36. Radhakrishnan K, Saxena S, Jillapalli R, et al. Barriers to and facilitators of South Asian Indian-Americans' engagement in advanced care planning behaviors. J Nurs Scholarsh 2017;49:294–302.
37. Worth A, Irshad T, Bhopal R, et al. Vulnerability and access to care for South Asian Sikh and Muslim patients with life limiting illness in Scotland: prospective longitudinal qualitative study. BMJ 2009;338:b183.
38. Washington KT, Bickel-Swenson D, Stephens N. Barriers to hospice use among African Americans: a systematic review. Health Soc Work 2008;33:267–74.

39. Jenkins C, Lapelle N, Zapka JG, et al. End-of-life care and African Americans: voices from the community. J Palliat Med 2005;8:585–92.
40. Braun KL, Karel H, Zir A. Family response to end-of-life education: differences by ethnicity and stage of caregiving. Am J Hosp Palliat Care 2006;23:269–76.
41. Elk R, Emanuel L, Hauser J, et al. Developing and Testing the Feasibility of a Culturally Based Tele-Palliative Care Consult Based on the Cultural Values and Preferences of Southern, Rural African American and White Community Members: A Program by and for the Community. Health Equity 2020;4:52–83.
42. Sudore RL, Lum HD, You JJ, et al. Defining advance care planning for adults: a consensus definition from a multidisciplinary delphi panel. J Pain Symptom Manage 2017;53:821–832 e1.

The Role of Informed Consent in Clinical and Research Settings

Essa Hariri, MD, MS[a,1], Mazen Al Hammoud, BS[b,1],
Erin Donovan, PhD[c], Kevin Shah, MD[d],
Michelle M. Kittleson, MD, PhD[e,*]

KEYWORDS

- Informed consent • Capacity • Competence • Autonomy
- Patient-physician relationship • Decision-making • Health care communication

KEY POINTS

- Informed consent is grounded in the principles of autonomy and respect involving a mutual understanding of the diagnosis, available treatment options, and consequences of opting for these different options.
- Informed consent should be provided by a capacitated patient or their proxy except for life-threatening emergencies where seeking consent would delay necessary treatment.
- For informed consent to be legally and ethically valid, patients must receive the necessary disclosures for decision-making, voluntarily give consent, and comprehend the information being communicated.
- Educational barriers, changing demographics, and advances in data technology are some of the most pressing challenges encountered during the process of obtaining informed consent.

Every human being of adult years and sound mind has a right to determine what shall be done with his own body; and a surgeon who performs an operation without his patient's consent commits an assault, for which he is liable in damages.

[a] Department of Internal Medicine, Cleveland Clinic Foundation, 9500 Euclid Ave, G10 Clinic, Cleveland OH 44195, USA; [b] Gilbert and Rose-Marie Chagoury School of Medicine, Lebanese American University, P.O. Box 36, Byblos, Lebanon; [c] Department of Communication Studies, The University of Texas at Austin, 2504A Whitis Ave, Austin, TX 78712, USA; [d] Department of Medicine, Division of Cardiology, University of Utah Hospital, 30 North 1900 East, Rm 4A100, Salt Lake City, UT 84132, USA; [e] Department of Cardiology, Smidt Heart Institute, Cedars-Sinai, Medical Center, 8670 Wilshire Blvd, 2nd floor, Beverly Hills, CA 90211, USA
[1] Denotes equal contribution.
* Corresponding author. Cedars-Sinai Heart Institute, 8670 Wilshire Boulevard, 2nd Floor, Los Angeles, CA 90211.
E-mail address: mitchelle.kittleson@cshs.org

Med Clin N Am 106 (2022) 663–674
https://doi.org/10.1016/j.mcna.2022.01.008
0025-7125/22/© 2022 Elsevier Inc. All rights reserved.

—Justice Benjamin Cardozo, 1914

INTRODUCTION

Informed consent plays an integral role in the patient-physician relationship. In this article, the authors present the concept of informed consent in 4 parts. First, they provide a brief history of the genesis of informed consent in clinical and research settings. Second, they describe the assessment of patient's capacity, the necessary first step in the informed consent process. Third, they explain the process of obtaining valid informed consent. Finally, the major contemporary challenges to the informed consent process are presented.

History

The foundational concepts of the informed consent process in modern medicine date back to ancient Greece.[1] Some modern medical ethicists believe that ancient Greeks adopted a paternalistic approach to the patient-physician relationship, which entails making decisions without explicit patient consent. However, there is considerable evidence from Cos school around 400 BC including *On Ancient Medicine*, *The Sacred Disease*, *Aphorisms*, *On Wounds in the Head*, and *The Oath* that proves the contrary: ancient Greek physicians interacted with patients based on honesty and trust.[2]

Several cases in the last century have shaped current widespread adoption of informed consent as the only ethical standard of care for clinicians and researchers. **Fig. 1** summarizes 4 major cases that laid the legal foundation of informed consent in the United States.

Although these 4 cases established the importance of patients consenting to interventions by physicians, the notion "informed consent" as a legal duty was first mentioned in 1957 in *Salgo v. Leland Stanford Jr. University Board of Trustees*.[3] The patient in this case was left paralyzed after translumbar aortography. Because the surgeon did not inform the patient about the potential risks associated with aortography, a California Court of Appeals ruled for the patient. Although consent had been obtained, the doctor did not provide the patient with the necessary information needed to make a decision; the standard of informed consent had not been met.

Informed consent is also a cornerstone of ethical medical research. One major historical event that highlighted the dangers of unethical research conduct was the USPHS Syphilis Study at Tuskegee. In 1932, 600 men—399 with syphilis, 201

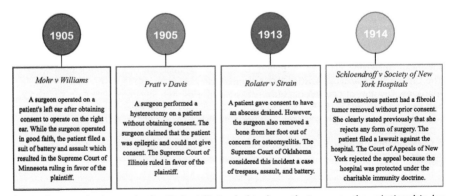

Fig. 1. Four seminal cases in the United States led to laws that govern the relationship between physicians and patients.

without—were enrolled in a natural history study.[4] By 1943, penicillin was the treatment of choice for syphilis, but the participants of that study were not informed that they had syphilis and were not offered treatment. This study highlights that informed consent is time specific (**Box 1**). Multiple advisory panels and governmental services have since condemned this unethical study and organized support for the study survivors and their families.

Another example of unethical research atrocities occurred during World War II, where German physicians conducted pseudoscientific medical experiments using thousands of concentration camp prisoners without their consent. In the 1947 Nuremberg Medical Trial, these doctors were indicted for their ruthless behavior, and 16 of 23 doctors were sentenced to death.[5]

The Nuremberg Trial resulted in the establishment of 10 principles for conducting research on human subjects which became the famous Nuremberg Code.[6] The Code's first principle is that "the voluntary consent of the human subject is absolutely essential." The Code also establishes that valid consent is voluntary, competent, informed, and comprehending. Following the Nuremberg Code, the Declaration of Helsinki was drafted to serve as a nonlegal guide to doctors in the conduct of ethical research.[7] Although there have been multiple revisions and controversies regarding the distinction between informed consent for therapeutic and nontherapeutic research, the Declaration provided early guidance for conduct on ethical research.

In 1938, the Federal Food, Drug, and Cosmetic Act[8] gave authority to the Food and Drug Administration (FDA) to oversee safety of food, drugs, medical devices, and cosmetics. In the United States in the 1960s, the FDA and the National Institutes of Health (NIH) established policies to protect human research subjects. In 1996, the FDA published the *Statement of Policy Concerning Consent for Use of Investigational New Drugs on Humans*,[9] inspired to a great extent by the Nuremberg Code and the Declaration of Helsinki.

Similar efforts were exerted by the NIH over this period, including the establishment of review boards that are now considered an integral part of the research process. In addition, the Department of Health and Human Services Office for the Protection of Research Risks oversees all federal agencies that conduct or support human subjects research under the Common Rule.

The past century has witnessed a dramatic transformation of the importance of informed consent and the regulation of research. This tightly regulated process is predicated on the value of individual autonomy and the patient's right to determine their medical fate.

Box 1
The two pillars of an informed consent

Informed consent is case specific.
- Informed consent given to perform a particular procedure does not automatically give consent to perform another intervention, even if the physician is operating in the patient's best interest.
- Two main scenarios would render this condition not applicable:
  - in cases of emergencies
  - when patients give a broad consent

Informed consent is time specific.
- Informed consent given for a particular procedure once does not automatically make it valid for later use.
- A patient's values and beliefs might change over time.

APPROACH: ASSESSMENT OF COMPETENCE AND CAPACITY

The informed consent process is grounded in principles of autonomy, respect, and good faith. Informed consent is not limited to a signed agreement to a particular treatment plan. Informed consent includes an understanding between physicians and their patients of the risks or consequences associated with a health care management plan or research-related activities. The first essential requirement of informed consent is a competent patient with the capacity to make decisions. Physicians must ensure that they are communicating with competent patients or competent proxies. The evaluation of a patient's mental capacity is necessary to balance respect for autonomy and protection of those with cognitive impairment.[10]

Competency Versus Capacity

Competency is a legal term that describes the mental capability to rationalize, understand one's circumstances, weigh risks and benefits, and voluntarily communicate a decision in a legal setting.[11] Capacity, on the other hand, is a functional determination that an individual is capable of making a medical decision within a given situation. The court is the only authority that can determine a patient's competency; however, not every case requires determination of competency from the court, as this would drain both the medical and judicial systems. Instead, physicians can evaluate a patient's capacity to make an informed consent.

Observational studies offer several predictors of incapacity.[10] Patients with dementia tend to have high rates of incapacity that is more pronounced with severe disease, as these patients suffer from progressive cognitive decline impairing their decision-making abilities.[12] Hospitalized patients with psychiatric disorders often demonstrate incompetency, most commonly those with acute schizophrenia compared with those with depression.[13,14] In these patients, lack of awareness and need for treatment of psychiatric disorders are the strongest predictors of incapacity.[15]

Conditions that limit cognition may also render patients incapacitated to make medical decisions, such as pharmacologic sedation or acute intoxication of an illicit substance. Medical conditions may also affect decision-making capacity, including unstable angina[16] or diabetic ketoacidosis.[17] As expected, incapacity is more apparent in inpatient settings,[18] with increasing age and cognitive impairment being the strongest predictors of mental incapacity.[19]

In a medical setting, physicians assume patients are competent unless they exhibit otherwise. This assumption is of practical importance, allowing health care professionals to focus on providing necessary diagnostic and therapeutic interventions without delay in patients who seem to have decision-making capacity on a standard initial evaluation.

Clinical Assessment of Capacity

When health care professionals suspect incapacity, they should perform a complete assessment to determine cognitive abilities and capacity to consent. The first step in evaluating capacity is to set the right climate (**Fig. 2**). Then, proceed to a clinical interview to assess its 4 criteria (**Fig. 3**). It is important in the case of an incapacitated patient to seek a surrogate decision-maker who may consent on behalf of the patient except in cases of life-threatening emergencies (**Boxes 2 and 3**).

Objective Tools for Cognition and Capacity

If there is a concern regarding the patient's cognition, formal cognition assessment may be performed.[20] There are several online tools for assessing cognition, including

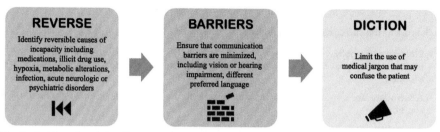

Fig. 2. Setting the right climate is the first step in evaluating capacity.

the Mini-Mental Status Examination (MMSE) and the Montreal Cognitive Assessment (MOCA). MMSE scores less than 20 to 24 increased the likelihood of incapacity by 6.3 times.[21] The MOCA questionnaire has 94% sensitivity and at least 90% specificity for detecting incapacity at a threshold score of 22.[22] If the assessment of capacity is still not clear, the use of systematic formal tools is indicated.[20] **Table 1** outlines a few examples of the most commonly used systematic approaches to capacity assessment. Of note, the major downside of these systematic tools is the significant time commitment involved to administer them, and for this reason, these tools are not often used in general practice but are more commonly used in clinical research.

THE INFORMED CONSENT PROCESS

After establishing the capacity of a patient or finding a surrogate in the case of an incapacitated patient, the next step is the informed consent process. Valid informed consent is based on a true understanding and clear physician-patient communication rather than just a signed form. In the Belmont Report,[23] the National Commission for the Protection of Human Subjects of Biomedical and Behavioral Research claims that the informed consent process is predicated on 3 foundational elements: information, voluntariness, and comprehension. These elements can occur in any order,

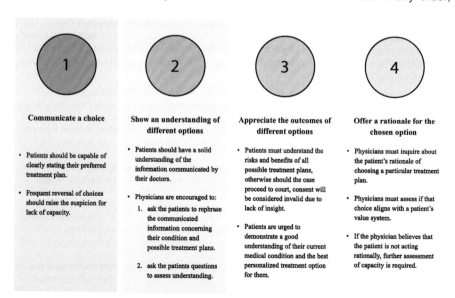

Fig. 3. The 4 commonly used clinical criteria to assess capacity.

Box 2
The role of the surrogate decision-maker

- Ethically and legally, valid informed consent must be given by a capacitated individual. If the patient does not have capacity to make decisions, a surrogate decision-maker must be assigned.
- A surrogate decision-maker becomes unnecessary during an emergency or life-threatening condition.
- If a patient does not have an authorized decision-maker, a family member or intimate associate may be considered per state laws or any individual who has a durable power of attorney.
- Physicians have a moral duty, to the best of their abilities, to ensure that the surrogate decision-maker is operating in the best interests of the patient and based on the patient's values.
- If the physician believes that the proxy is acting in bad faith, an ethics consultation may be required; legal consultation is usually a last resort.
- Physicians should inform conscious incapacitated patients about their plans and interventions even if consent is given by the surrogate decision-maker.

---

although it is customary to provide information, emphasize the voluntariness of the decision-making process, and then assess comprehension. The opportunity for voluntariness may vary depending on the urgency of the clinical situation, but clinicians should emphasize that patients may adjust their decision as they learn more about the indications, benefits, risks, and alternatives of a given intervention (**Fig. 4** and **Box 3**).

Box 3
Clinical case: information, voluntariness, and comprehension.

Sample Case
Mr M, a 76-year-old patient with a history of dementia, was rushed to the emergency department after a syncopal episode. After being resuscitated in the emergency room, his electrocardiogram revealed a third-degree AV block with a heart rate of 32 BPM and a blood pressure of 89/67 mm Hg. His physical examination, laboratory tests, and imaging results confirmed the need for a pacemaker implantation. How would you proceed with the process of obtaining informed consent?

Suggested approach with the patient (if has capacity) or the surrogate decision-maker
Disclosing medical information: "Your fainting spell occurred because your heart rate was too slow, which can happen with age. A pacemaker can be implanted to protect you from a low heart rate and prevent fainting spells. There are risks of infection, bleeding, and injury to blood vessels. However, the risks are small and without the pacemaker, you could suffer serious injury from future fainting spells."
Inquiring about patient preferences for information: "I can provide more detail about the reasons for pacemaker implantation and the benefits and risks of the procedure. What questions do you have?"
Emphasizing voluntariness: "While my medical recommendation is to proceed with a pacemaker, this is not an emergency. You are currently monitored and temporarily protected against episodes of low heart rate. We should decide within the next 1 to 2 days about whether or not you will have the pacemaker. Would you like to give this more thought and discuss more later today?"
Assessing comprehension: "To make sure I've explained this correctly, can you tell me the reason I am recommending a pacemaker? What about the risks of the procedure? What could happen if you decide not to have a pacemaker?"

Table 1
Commonly validated clinical assessment tools to assess capacity

Test	Authors & Date	Time to Administer	Patient Population	Capacity Criteria Assessed
Aid to Capacity Evaluation (ACE)	Etchells et al (1999)	10–20 min	Medical inpatients	Understanding, appreciation, and reasoning
Assessment of Consent Capacity for Treatment (ACT)	Cea and Fischer (2003)	45 min	Adults with or without mild-to-moderate mental retardation	Understanding, appreciation, reasoning, and communicating a choice
Hopkins Competency Test (HCAT)	Janofsky et al (1992)	10 min	Neuropsychiatric and medical inpatients; outpatients with psychotic disorders; patients with Alzheimer's disease; nursing home residents.	Understanding
MacArthur Competence Assessment Tool for Treatment (MacCAT-T)	Grisso and Appelbaum 1998)	15–20 min	Medical inpatients	Understanding, appreciation, reasoning, and communicating a choice

Information	Comprehension
The physician's role is to:	• Assess the patient's comprehension in four core elements:

• Accurately and sensitively disclose the diagnosis, nature and purpose of recommended interventions, burdens, risks, and expected benefits of all options including forgoing treatment, and any medical errors.	- Risks
	   - Benefits
	   - Alternatives

• Inquire about the patient's specific preferences to receive certain medical information before it is available, and tailor disclosure of information appropriately.	- General knowledge about the procedure or treatment • Avoid focusing only on risks, which is a physician-centered approach.
- respect patient's wishes including not wanting to receive specific medical information	• The teach-back method is a validated method to assess patient's understanding.
- consult patient's family, colleagues, or an ethics committee to assess the relative benefits and harms associated with delaying communication of information based on the patient's preferences	• asking open-ended questions allows patients to rephrase or explain the information communicated to them in their own way
• Document the informed consent conversation in the medical record.	• it evaluates patient's understanding as well as the physician's ability to communicate complex information
Voluntariness	• it improves disease knowledge, patient satisfaction, medication adherence, quality of life
• Patients may withdraw written or verbal informed consent at any point.	• it is recommended by the American Heart Association and the American Diabetes Association
• Giving patients time to consider options before proceeding with a particular plan reinforces the validity of the informed consent.	
• Document any withdrawal request in writing including date, time, and relevant circumstances.	

Fig. 4. The foundational elements of informed consent.

Informed Consent for Research

Although the foundational concepts of the informed consent process in research settings are similar to those in clinical settings, the former requires a higher standard of consent because the patient would be susceptible to the risks of unapproved interventions.[24] Participants in clinical research should provide informed consent after the full disclosure of necessary information.[7] This information includes a written summary of the study design along with possible consequences of the tested intervention or the control group in understandable language.

The institutional review board (IRB) provides legal protection to human research subjects involved in clinical research. The IRB is governed by the Code of Federal Regulations Title 21, Part 45 (21 CFR 56).[25] The main roles of the IRB are to verify that valid informed consent was obtained, ensure that the potential benefits of the research exceeds the possible risks, and protect participants' integrity and autonomy.[24] In addition, the NIH Office for Human Research Protection issues guidelines on protecting human subjects involved in federally funded research. Nevertheless, the current standard of practice in clinical research is far from the theoretic ideal.[24] Some researchers may use complex documents in the consent process with legal and medical jargon to minimize their risk of exposure to litigation.

FUTURE DIRECTIONS

There is a well-documented gap between the current application of the informed consent process and the ideal theoretic framework that promotes patient's autonomy and bodily integrity.[26] Many challenges arise during the consent process between a physician or investigator and the patient or study participant. Some of the most pressing challenges encountered during this process include (1) educational barriers, (2) changing demographics, and (3) advances in data technology.

Educational Barriers

A patient's or a research participant's literacy level largely influences the effectiveness of the consent process, and educational barriers limit the comprehension of consent information.[27] In a survey of 100 IRB-approved consent forms, investigators found that consent forms were relatively long with a mean readability of Grade 11.6,[28] which is of significant concern, as the reading level of an average American layperson is grade 6 to 8.[29] Furthermore, in the United States, more than one-third of adults have basic or below basic health literacy[30] and around half of the US population have basic or below basic quantitative literacy, making the proper understanding of numerical data and statistics challenging.[30] Even though the Code of Federal Regulations states that consent information should be presented in an understandable language to the patient or study participant (21 CFR 50.20), a study at 2 urban US hospitals including 2659 patients reported that 59.5% could not understand a standard informed consent document.[18,31] Furthermore, another study of informed consent forms adopted by 5 of the largest national cancer clinical trial groups found that the forms were "slightly less difficult to read and understand than medical journals, but substantially more difficult than materials from the popular press."[32]

Because comprehension is an essential component of the consent process, consent given by a patient who does not understand the communicated information is not valid. Furthermore, people who have lower health literacy are particularly vulnerable because they are least able to acknowledge what they do not know and are the least likely to ask questions.[33]

There are strategies to address these issues. In a randomized study of 1500 participants, multimedia aids including simplified language and visual representations improved the informed consent process,[34] and interactive interventions, including multimedia aids such as short clips or infographics demonstrating particular interventions or challenging medical concepts, may be superior to noninteractive interventions.[35] Test/feedback and teach-back techniques, along with bidirectional communication, can improve the consent process. Although most informed consent interventions focus on supplementing patients' understanding with additional materials, improving consent should focus on better communication, not just more information. Even patients with adequate reading skills and high health literacy prefer consent materials that are easy to navigate.[36]

Changing Demographics

Another major contemporary barrier to a successful and effective informed consent process is changing demographics. The US population is becoming older and more ethnically diverse.[26] The increase in awareness of the need to address social determinants of health and health inequity is apparent in the medical community, and approaches to informed consent should be tailored for different ethnicities and minority groups. It is thus essential to amend guidelines detailing the process of informed consent to embrace cultural diversity and prepare the new generation of physicians by developing comprehensive training programs that promote cultural intelligence.[37] Furthermore, the next few decades will experience a doubling in the percentage of people older than 65 years and an even larger increase in the percentage of people older than 85 years.[26] The number of patients with Alzheimer disease is expected to double by 2050.[38] As such, the proportion of adult patients who are deemed incompetent for their own decision-making is likely to increase over time. It is crucial to prepare health care professionals to assess capacity in an effective and systematic manner. Besides training health care professionals, ethical and medical societies should unify guidelines that would allow physicians to involve trusted family members and friends in the decision-making process.[26]

Advances in Data Technology

Advanced technologies and artificial intelligence generate data that could be used for many purposes. These technologies raise challenging ethical questions. For example, next-generation sequencing generates an unprecedented amount of data in both clinical and research settings. These data allow not only identification of the patient or research participant but also blood relatives.[26] Hence, providing consent for genomic sequence analysis involves more than individual autonomy per se.

Another challenge of data technology is related to biobanks containing information on patients' vital signs or biological materials. The data stored in a biobank could be used at any time for any purpose and by different investigators. For instance, data gathered from Apple watches for the Apple Heart Study[39] are subject to unclear consent processes that many users sign without reviewing the extent of those consents. Informed consent in these scenarios is no longer case- and time-specific, which can jeopardize patient's autonomy and integrity.

DISCUSSION

There are nuances when addressing informed consent in one's practice. These nuances mainly stem from the need to highly personalize informed consent processes for every patient. The need for informed consent has been codified to highlight fundamental human rights including autonomy and integrity. The modern process of informed consent is thus regarded as a legal obligation rather than an ethical duty toward patients. Medical societies should invest in decision-making algorithms that could guide physicians' thought processes. The challenge is in providing a standardized decision-making framework that offers a certain degree of flexibility to tailor the informed consent process to every patient. The advent of artificial intelligence and machine learning allows new opportunities for the development of reliable algorithms that could provide tailorized decision-making guidance for every scenario.

SUMMARY

Informed consent is an integral component of any clinical or research interaction with patients. The process of informed consent has evolved over the past century through numerous lessons learned from malpractice and unethical conduct of human research. Understanding the historical and legal framework of informed consent, as well as the process of obtaining valid consent, is crucial to navigate through current challenges brought on by educational barriers, changing demographics, and advances in data technology. In this data-driven era, bioethicists, legal advocates, and health care professionals need to modernize the informed consent process. Regardless of future challenges, the priority will always remain the same: informed consent is more than just a signed form. Informed consent is based on true understanding and clear physician-patient communication and strives to preserve patients' autonomy and integrity.

CLINICS CARE POINTS

- The most important first step in informed consent is assessing capacity.
- If a patient lacks capacity, identify a surrogate decision-maker.
- When obtaining informed consent, deliver adequate information, assure patient's comprehension, and assure patient's voluntariness in providing or withdrawing consent.
- Informed consent is the foundation of ethical conduct of clinical research, and engaging the Institutional Review Board is an essential step toward that goal.
- Consider developing or supporting development of guidelines to mitigate contemporary challenges to informed consent including meeting the complex needs of the aging population and comfortably managing large volumes of stored data from artificial intelligence and biobanks.

DISCLAIMERS

The authors do not have any relevant disclosures.

REFERENCES

1. Murray PM. The History of Informed Consent. Iowa Orthop J 1990;10:104–9.
2. Miles SH. Hippocrates and informed consent. Lancet 2009;374(9698):1322–3.
3. Salgo v. Leland Stanford etc. Bd. Trustees, 317 P.2d 170, 154 Cal. App. 2d 560, 154 Cal. 2d 560 (Ct. App.1957).
4. McCallum JM, Arekere DM, Green BL, et al. Awareness and Knowledge of the U.S. Public Health Service Syphilis Study at Tuskegee: Implications for Biomedical Research. J Health Care Poor Underserved 2006;17(4):716.
5. Wright Q. The Law of the Nuremberg Trial. Am J Int Law 1947;41(1):38–72.
6. Katz J. The Nuremberg Code and the Nuremberg Trial: A Reappraisal. J Am Med Assoc 1996;276(20):1662–6.
7. Association WM. World Medical Association Declaration of Helsinki: Ethical Principles for Medical Research Involving Human Subjects. J Am Med Assoc 2013; 310(20):2191–4.
8. Cavers David F. The Food, Drug, and Cosmetic Act of 1938: its legislative history and its substantive provisions. Law & Contemp. Probs 1939;6.
9. Goddard JI. Consent for use of investigational new drugs on humans: statement of policy by the food and drug administration. J New Drugs 1966;6(6):366–7.
10. Appelbaum PS. Assessment of Patients' Competence to Consent to Treatment. N Engl J Med 2007;357(18):1834–40.
11. Buchanan A. Mental capacity, legal competence and consent to treatment. J R Soc Med 2004;97(9):415–20.
12. Kim Scott YH, HT Karlawish Jason, Caine Eric D. Current state of research on decision-making competence of cognitively impaired elderly persons. Am J Geriatr Psychiatry 2002;151–65.
13. Appelbaum PS. The MacArthur Treatment Competence Study. III: abilities of patients to consent to psychiatric and medical treatments. Law Hum Behav 1995;149–74.
14. Vollmann J, Bauer A, Danker-Hopfe H, et al. Competence of mentally ill patients: a comparative empirical study. Psychol Med 2003;33(8):1463–71.
15. Cairns R, Maddock C, Buchanan A, et al. Prevalence and predictors of mental incapacity in psychiatric in-patients. Br J Psychiatry : J Ment Sci 2005;187: 379–85.
16. Appelbaum PS, Grisso T. Capacities of Hospitalized, Medically Ill Patients to Consent to Treatment. Psychosomatics 1997;38(2):119–25.
17. Palmer BW, Dunn LB, Appelbaum PS, et al. Assessment of Capacity to Consent to Research Among Older Persons With Schizophrenia, Alzheimer Disease, or Diabetes Mellitus: Comparison of a 3-Item Questionnaire With a Comprehensive Standardized Capacity Instrument. Arch Gen Psychiatry 2005;62(7):726–33.
18. Stanley Barbara, et al. The elderly patient and informed consent: empirical findings. JAMA 1984;252(10):1302–1306.
19. Raymont V, Bingley W, Buchanan A, et al. Prevalence of mental incapacity in medical inpatients and associated risk factors: cross-sectional study. Lancet 2004;364(9443):1421–7.
20. Barstow C, Shahan B, Roberts M. Evaluating Medical Decision-Making Capacity in Practice. Am Fam Physician 2018;98(1):40–6.

21. Sessums LL, Zembrzuska H, Jackson JL. Does This Patient Have Medical Decision-Making Capacity? JAMA 2011;306(4):420–7.

22. Karlawish J, Cary M, Moelter ST, et al. Cognitive impairment and PD patients' capacity to consent to research. Neurology 2013;81(9):801.

23. Miracle Vickie A. The Belmont Report: The triple crown of research ethics. Dimensions of Critical Care, Nursing 2016;35(4):223–228.

24. Bernat JL. Informed consent. Muscle & Nerve 2001;24(5):614–21.

25. US Food and Drug Administration. CFR-code of federal regulations title 2017;21.

26. Grady Christine. Enduring and emerging challenges of informed consent. N Engl J Med 2015;372(9):855–62.

27. Raich PC, Plomer KD, Coyne CA. Literacy, Comprehension, and Informed Consent in. Clin Res 2001;19(4):437–45.

28. Larson E, Foe G, Lally R. Reading Level and Length of Written Research Consent Forms. Clin Translational Sci 2015;8(4):355–6.

29. Foe Gabriella, Elaine L. Larson. "Reading level and comprehension of research consent forms: An integrative review. J Empirical Res Hum Res Ethics 2016; 11(1):31–46.

30. Kutner M, Greenburg E, Jin Y, et al., The Health Literacy of America's Adults: Results from the 2003 National Assessment of Adult Literacy. NCES 2006-483, 2006, National Center for education statistics.

31. Williams Mv, Parker RM, Baker DW, et al. Inadequate Functional Health Literacy Among Patients at Two Public Hospitals. J Am Med Assoc 1995;274(21): 1677–82.

32. Morrow GR. How Readable Are Subject Consent Forms? J Am Med Assoc 1980; 244(1):56–8.

33. Donovan-Kicken E, Mackert M, Guinn TD, et al. Health Literacy, Self-Efficacy, and Patients' Assessment of Medical Disclosure and Consent Documentation. Health Commun 2012;27(6):581–90.

34. Kraft SA, Constantine M, Magnus D, et al. A randomized study of multimedia informational aids for research on medical practices: Implications for informed consent 2016;14(1):94–102.

35. Glaser J, Nouri S, Fernandez A, et al. Interventions to Improve Patient Comprehension in Informed Consent for Medical and Surgical Procedures: An Updated Systematic Review. Rev Med Decis Making 2020;(2):119–43.

36. Donovan EE, Crook B, Brown LE, et al. An Experimental Test of Medical Disclosure and Consent Documentation: Assessing Patient Comprehension, Self-Efficacy, and Uncertainty. Commun Monogr 2014;81(2):239–60.

37. Ekmekci PE, Arda B. Interculturalism and Informed Consent: Respecting Cultural Differences without Breaching Human Rights. Cultura (Iasi, Romania) 2017; 14(2):159.

38. Hebert Liesi E, et al. Alzheimer disease in the United States (2010–2050) estimated using the 2010 census. Neurology 2013;80(19):1778–83.

39. Perez MV, et al. Large-scale assessment of a smartwatch to identify atrial fibrillation. N Engl J Med 2019;381(20):1909–17.

Classifying and Disclosing Medical Errors

Maria Barsky, MD[a],*, Andrew P.J. Olson, MD[b,c], Gopi J. Astik, MD MS[d]

KEYWORDS

- Medical error • Patient harm • Disclosure • Error disclosure • Health communication

KEY POINTS

- Medical errors are common and include adverse events, delays in care, near misses, delays in diagnosis, and unanticipated outcomes.
- Harm from medical error is classified as potential or actual harm, and graded in severity from no harm to death.
- Medical errors cause significant harm to patients and their families, including physical and emotional harm.
- Disclosing medical errors minimizes perceived harm of error by patients, decreases litigation, and rebuilds trust between provider and patient.
- Error disclosure should contain facts and an apology.

INTRODUCTION

The 2016 report in British Medical Journal found medical errors to be the third leading cause of death in the United States, which is shocking, yet not surprising.[1] The actual number of deaths attributable to medical errors is controversial, but it is accepted that medical errors are common.[2] Medical professionals should be able to understand what medical errors are, why they occur, and how they affect patients. Disclosing diagnostic and treatment errors to patients is crucial in minimizing the perceived harm of medical errors by patients as well as creating a culture of openness, learning,

[a] Hospitalist Program, UC Irvine Medical Center, 101 The City Drive South, Suite 500, Orange, CA 92868, USA; [b] Section of Hospital Medicine, Division of General Internal Medicine, Department of Medicine, , University of Minnesota Medical School, 420 Delaware Street Southeast, MMC 741, Minneapolis, MN 55455, USA; [c] Division of Pediatric Hospital Medicine, Department of Pediatrics, University of Minnesota Medical School, 420 Delaware Street Southeast, MMC 741, Minneapolis, MN 55455, USA; [d] Division of Hospital Medicine, Northwestern University Feinberg School of Medicine, 251 East Huron Street Suite 16-738, Chicago, IL 60611, USA
* Corresponding author.
E-mail address: mbarsky@uci.edu
Twitter: @BarskyMasha (M.B.); @andrewolsonmd (A.P.J.O.); @gopiastik (G.J.A.)

Med Clin N Am 106 (2022) 675–687
https://doi.org/10.1016/j.mcna.2022.02.007
0025-7125/22/Published by Elsevier Inc.

medical.theclinics.com

and coproduction of health. Although disclosing medical errors to patients is critical, unfortunately many clinicians do not feel trained in the ability to have these conversations.[3].In this article, we explore medical errors and their disclosure: their definition, the harms they cause, their perception by patients and loved ones, why disclosure is important, and best practices for disclosure.

DEFINITIONS
Medical Errors

In the 1950s, medical errors were largely considered a necessary evil of modern medical advancement and there was little research on the matter.[4] In the past several decades, however, there has been substantial research on medical errors. This research has, not surprisingly, found that medical errors are not only detrimental to the patient, but costly to the medical system.[5] Medical error is a broad term that encompasses several entities: adverse events, near misses, delays in care and diagnoses, and unanticipated outcomes. Here, we review some key literature regarding the definition of medical errors.

In the 1990s, the Harvard Medical Practice Study, the Quality in Australian Health Study, and the Utah Colorado Medical Practice Study gave prominence to the term "adverse event." These foundational studies developed and validated methods for defining and measuring errors while also raising the visibility of the topic in high-profile, well-respected journals. The Harvard Medical Practice and the Utah Colorado Medical Practice Studies defined an adverse event as an unintended injury to patients caused by medical management—rather than the underlying condition of the patient—that results in measurable disability, prolonged hospitalization, or both.[6–8] The Australian Health Study defined an adverse event as an unintended injury or complication that results in disability, death, or prolonged hospital stay and is caused by health care management rather than the patients' disease.[9,10] Importantly, this definition includes acts of omission—failing to do the right thing—as well as acts of commission—doing something wrong—when exploring failures of health care.

The authors of these landmark studies clarify—importantly—that adverse events due to medical error are preventable. They went on to qualify preventable events as events that occurred because of failure to follow accepted medical practice.[11] A subset of preventable adverse events is negligent adverse events, which satisfy the legal criteria determining negligence. Negligence is care that falls below the standard expected of physicians in their community.[7,8] The final category of adverse events is ameliorable adverse events, which are events that are not preventable, but the severity of the injury could have been reduced if different actions or procedures had been performed or followed.[12]

Not all medical errors lead to adverse events: those errors that occur without causing an adverse event are "near misses." Near misses often unmask or are a harbinger of unsafe situations and are indistinguishable from a preventable adverse event, except for the final outcome.[11] James Reason's "Swiss cheese" model describes how errors eventually lead to adverse events: they are not caught in the multiple layers of defense of our medical system.[13,14] Another medical error that does not always lead to an adverse event is a delay in diagnosis or care. A delay in diagnosis that does not lead to an adverse event can still be considered a medical error, however. Finally, an unanticipated outcome is one that differs from an expected result and, if preventable, can be considered a medical error. **Table 1** provides a summary of the terms associated with medical errors and delivers examples for each definition.

Table 1
Definitions and examples of terms associated with medical error

Term	Definition	Example
Preventable adverse event	Adverse event that that occurred due to failure to follow accepted medical practice (at the current level of average practitioner that manages the disease in question)	A physician starts a patient with a documented history of penicillin allergy on penicillin, leading to anaphylaxis.
Ameliorable adverse event	Adverse events that are not preventable, but the severity of injury could have been reduced if different actions or procedures had been performed or followed	A patient is placed on furosemide for heart failure exacerbation without a clear follow-up plan and returns to the hospital with hypokalemia.
Near miss	Unsafe situations and are indistinguishable from a preventable adverse event, except for the outcome	A doctor prescribes the wrong dose of drug, but the error is caught by the pharmacist before the drug is administered.
Delay in diagnosis/care	Nonoptimal interval of time between the onset of symptoms, identification, and initiation of treatment	A 50-year-old man's complaints of new severe headaches were dismissed as migraines until final diagnosis of glioblastoma.
Unanticipated outcomes	Outcome that differs from an expected result	A patient has persistent leakage of ascites after paracentesis. No medical error occurred if all standards were followed, such as creation of z-track.
Omission leading to medical error	Medical error that occurs because the physician or medical system failed to do the right thing	An inpatient physician forgets to order a vital medication that a patient is on at home that leads to an adverse event.
Commission leading to medical error	Medical error that occurs because the physician or medical system did something wrong	A physician orders the wrong medication with a similar name for the patient, which leads to an adverse event.

Harm

Defining harm from medical error can be challenging. In this section, we review some validated tools for assessing the harm associated with medical errors as well as some common themes and challenges in defining harm. Some examples of harm classifications and scales include the Medication Error and Risk Assessment Index (NCC-MERP),[15] The Harm Associated with Medication Error Classification (HAMEC classification),[16] the World Health Organization (WHO) harm classification,[17] Agency for Healthcare Research and Quality Healthcare Associated Preventable Harm (HARM scale),[18] and the American Society of Healthcare and Risk Management (ASHRM) harm scale.[19] As harm is an outcome, it can be challenging to clearly link harm with process, especially as there are varying and valid patient and physician perspectives whether the harm is tied to a medical error and to the medical event.

All harm classification tools assess if there was potential or actual preventable harm associated with the error. If actual harm occurred, the severity of the harm is then determined. The ASHRM harm scale suggests first determining if there is a deviation in standard practice. If there was a deviation from practice, then preventable harm occurred.[19] In most health systems, interdisciplinary panels determine if actual harm or a near miss (potential harm) occurred. Actual harm occurs when the medical error reaches the patient.[16] Overall, both near misses and errors that cause harm are rated in severity of the harm caused or that could have occurred.[16,19]

There are several scales that classify harm severity for medical errors. One example is the 2012 HARM scale, which uses a two-part assessment of harm and asks the user the degree of harm on a 5-point scale with 3 categories between no harm and death and then indicates separately the duration of harm.[18] ASHRM[19] used the HARM tool as a basis for a more comprehensive harm classification tool. The WHO developed a similar scale ranging from "no harm" to "death" with levels such as mild, moderate, severe, and death.[17] The HAMEC classification is a new tool that was proposed in 2019.[16] This scale uses potential and actual harm, as well as the severity of harm. One of the most established harm classification tools pertaining to medication errors is the NCC-MERP. The NCC-MERP uses a letter system to score the severity of actual harm or potential harm caused.[15] **Table 2** summarizes some available harm scales.

CURRENT EVIDENCE: THE PATIENT EXPERIENCE

Thus far, we have discussed the definition of medical error and harm but have not delved into the most tangible and painful real-world consequences of medical error: the hurt experienced by patients and their families. The literature surrounding the patient experience of harm and error is expanding, yet continues to lag behind the literature describing prevalence, causes, and mitigation strategies for errors and adverse events. Many of the existing studies of patient experience of errors and harm have small sample sizes or include only those patients who are planning legal action; a small and biased sample, as most errors do not lead to malpractice action.[20] Here we review the research into the perceptions of error by patients and families.

A study by Mazor and colleagues in 2009 used an in-depth interview process to understand the ramifications of medical error on patients and their families.[20] These interviews were later reviewed by physicians to determine if an error occurred, if there was a possible error, or if there was an unanticipated outcome without evidence of the error. The study yielded major themes and subthemes related to patient and family experience of medical errors).

Interestingly, most errors in this study were not disclosed by the primary provider. Not only does this study demonstrate the broad impact medical errors have on patients but it also highlights that not disclosing medical errors does not necessarily result in less detection of errors by patients. In fact, lack of communication can lead patients and family members to a false conclusion that a medical error did occur. For example, if a poor clinical outcome occurs despite the provision of standard medical care, a family or patient could surmise that an error occurred when it did not.

A survey of patients in Alberta examined the perception of quality of the health care system, frequency of preventable medical error, responsibility for preventable medical error, as well as causes and solutions to reduce preventable medical errors.[21] Respondents who had personal experience with preventable medical errors were more pessimistic about the frequency of preventable medical errors, the transparency of reporting, and were less satisfied with the health care services they receive. Most respondents found fault with individual clinicians more than the health care system. Respondents suggested that health care professionals can increase public satisfaction and confidence by admitting errors to patients, taking more time with patients, caring more, and communicating more carefully. Most respondents agreed that

Table 2
Examples of harm rating scales

Scale	Grading System of Actual Harm	Grading System of Potential Harm
HARM[18] Healthcare-Associated Preventable Harm Classification	*Death* *Severe*/permanent or temporary harm; symptomatic; requires life-saving intervention *Moderate* harm/permanent or temporary; symptomatic; requires intervention *Mild*/temporary or no harm; symptomatic; minimal or no intervention required	*No detectable harm*/no harm; asymptomatic Almost happened
HAMEC[16] The Harm Associated with Medication Error Classification	*0. No harm,* no harm or change in monitoring *1. Minor,* non-life-threatening, temporary harm. Minimal increase in length of stay (<1 day). *2. Moderate,* minor non-life-threatening, temporary harm that would require assessment to a change in patient condition or monitoring. *3. Serious,* major, non-life-threatening, temporary harm that would require high level of care or increase LOS >1 day *4. Severe,* life-threatening or mortal harm, or major permanent harm; may require high level of care or increased LOS > 1 day.	*0. No harm,* no potential harm or change in monitoring: *1. Minor,* potential for minor, non-life-threatening, temporary harm; minimal increase in length of stay (<1 day). *2. Moderate,* potential for minor non-life-threatening, temporary harm that would require assessment to a change in patient condition or monitoring. *3. Serious,* potential for major, non-life-threatening, temporary harm that would require high level of care or increase LOS >1 day *4. Severe,* potential for life-threatening or mortal harm, or major permanent harm. May require high level of care or increased LOS > 1 day.
NCC-MERP[15] NCC MERP Definition of a Medication Error and Risk Assessment Index	Error—Harm *E*: An error occurred, resulting in treatment or intervention *F*: An error occurred, resulting in prolonged hosptitalization and caused temporary harm *G*: An error occurred that caused permanent harm to the patient *H*: An error occurred that resulted in near-death *I*: Event resulted in death	*A*: No error—circumstances or events that have the capacity to cause harm Error—no harm *B*: Error occurred, but medication did not reach the patient *C*: Error occurred and reached the patient but did not cause harm *D*: Error occurred and reached the patient and did not cause harm but required extra monitoring

physicians should be required to report medical errors. The study's findings were similar to those of Blendon and colleagues in the United States, although US residents believe medical errors happen more often than Canadians.[22]

A study from 1986 to 1989 by Hickson and colleagues explored why some families of children that experience a medical error choose to file malpractice claims.[23] The study found that common reasons were advice from others, financial hardship, and the perception that there was a cover-up of the error.[23] Multiple studies show that inadequate delivery of information and negative interactions with the provider are leading causes of increased litigious intentions.[24,25] Duclos and colleagues found that not only does an acknowledgment of error decrease frustrations for patients and families but also that patients who had received some sort of communication and acknowledgment of the error were more likely to have an ongoing relationship with the provider and were more likely to perceive "no fault" in the event.[26] The same study uncovered that quick action must be taken to rectify the mistake and an answer provided to the following questions: "What happened?," "What is next?," and "Is it fixable?"[26] Schwappach and Koeck found that the severity of the error was the most important factor in patient perception followed by honest disclosure of the error by physicians.[27]

CLINICAL RELEVANCE

Recognizing that an error occurred is only part of the process. An equally important domain is the effective disclosure of such errors to patients and their families. Disclosure of medical error is paramount for ethical reasons as well as maintaining patients' safety and patients' trust in the medical system. In this section, we summarize the importance of disclosing medical errors.

Ethics

The basic ethical principles that traditionally guide medical care include patient autonomy, justice, veracity, fidelity, beneficence, and nonmaleficence. Disclosure of medical error can be tied to each of these principles. Patient autonomy is a principle that describes patients' right to make choices about their lives and their care. Disclosing medical errors allows patients to make informed choices about the next steps in their care and who will oversee their future care in the context of this error. Failure to disclose the medical error robs the patient of this participation in their own medical care. The principle of justice is also deeply connected to medical error disclosure, with the emphasis on transparency. Perhaps the most obviously relatable ethical principle to error disclosure is veracity, or truth telling—which is essentially the definition of medical error disclosure. Fidelity, or patients' trust centered on the provider doing what they said they would do, cannot coexist with deceit or deception. Legal self-interest may need to be curtailed by the principle of fidelity. Beneficence is the concept of "doing good" or acting in accordance with the patient's welfare. Disclosing medical errors allows for the next steps to be taken to maximize patient's well-being posterror and doing good for future patients. For example, disclosing an original delay in cancer diagnosis can prompt a more expedited workup. Finally, nonmaleficence, or the concept of doing "no harm" can also be extended to minimizing harm. Prompt disclosure of an error, if harm occurred, can minimize further harm or identify possibilities for future harm.[28] The medical community is in full agreement that disclosure of medical error is the ethically right thing to do, although there are distinct perceived and actual barriers to doing so.

Standard Response to Errors

An important part of patient safety is the transparent response to errors.[29] All errors should be reported to both patients and the local institutional authority. An example of such reporting is when an error occurs related to medication dosage, the patient is made aware, and the incident is reported to the hospital patient safety team to review the incident and prevent it from happening again. Patients want a clear apology with an expression of empathy, disclosure of harmful errors along with errors that may not be apparent to them, followed by an investigation into the root cause of the error.[20,30] A multidisciplinary review of the error by all personnel involved—directly or indirectly—should involve an analysis of factors that led to the event. A thorough reflection on factors causing the error should frame a discussion on how to prevent similar errors in the future.[31] A follow-up discussion with patients should also include prevention strategies discussed during the evaluation of the error. Only through a process of disclosure of medical error—both to the institution and patient—can the necessary steps be taken to prevent further harm to the particular patient who experienced the event and to future patients.

Approach to Disclosing Errors

Disclosing errors to patients is of the utmost importance and many medical centers have disclosure policies that aim to improve transparency.[32] Discussing errors and harm with patients should be done in an open and honest way with a focus on patient safety. Often, clinicians themselves should be the ones to discuss errors with patients to provide information, support, and answer questions. To do this, clinicians must be trained in how to effectively disclose and should also be provided support by the institution before and after the event and disclosure.[33] It is also important to ensure that trainees are not tasked with error disclosure on their own without the support of their clinical supervisors, as this is inappropriate from both an educational and patient care perspective. Furthermore, it is fundamental to support clinicians during this disclosure process and provide ongoing emotional support even after the error is disclosed.

Guidelines for disclosure of errors involve a frank conversation with plain language referring to the incident as an error, providing necessary details, and an honest apology.[34,35] These conversations begin by clearly stating there was an error. They then describe the course of events, using nontechnical language. Next, the nature of the mistake, consequences, and the corrective action are all discussed. Clinicians must avoid speculation about the causative factors leading to the error, blaming other clinicians, and promising actions that may not be realistic. Importantly, the disclosure must contain an apology. The discussion should not be defensive nor a statement of regret but should provide objective facts along with a clear apology *as a means of empathic human connection*. Then, elicit questions or concerns and address them. Finally, plan the next steps and next contact with the patient in very clear, discrete terms. After the initial conversation, it is important to follow words with action. This includes minimizing further harm to the patient, financial compensation to the family if appropriate, and making institutional changes to prevent future similar events. **Table 3** and **Box 1** summarize best practice for disclosing medical errors.

Along with disclosing the error to the patient, it is important for the multidisciplinary team involved in the care of the patient to debrief on the event. Not only is this debriefing cathartic but it also allows evaluation into the event from multiple perspectives.

Disclosing medical errors made by others may be tricky. In general, all clinicians involved in error who had direct patient contact should be present for disclosure, including comanaging physicians and trainees. If there was a lack of supervision of

Table 3
Best practice principles in communicating medical errors with examples

Principle	Example
Begin by stating there has been an error	"I am sorry to say that there was a misdiagnosis regarding your lung mass. It is not pneumonia, like I thought, but lung cancer."
Describe the course of events using nontechnical language	"As you recall, you saw four months ago with a new cough, and we performed a chest x-ray that showed an area of concern for what looked to me like pneumonia. The radiologist also thought that it was either pneumonia or a lung mass,(possibly cancer). When you returned 2 weeks ago with the cough, we got a CT which showed the same concerning area but now larger. Ultimately, you received a biopsy that confirmed the diagnosis of lung cancer."
State the nature of the mistake, consequences, and corrective action	"The mistake was a delay in diagnosis that may have led to the progression of the cancer. We now plan to complete all the scans necessary to see if there is indeed progression and initiate treatment as soon as possible."
Express personal regret and apologize	"I am truly sorry that I caused a delay in your care and diagnosis."
Elicit questions or concerns and address them	"I know this is a lot to take in. What questions can I help answer?"
Plan the next step and next contact with patient	"We will perform a PET-CT in two days, and we will schedule an appointment in four days when the results have returned."
Debriefing and multidisciplinary analysis	A debriefing session in a multidisciplinary team can further decide if RCA needs to be done, as well as potential ways to prevent further errors. In this case, the clinic can decide to have the radiologist forward all results to the provider when a final read is available, and guidelines can be provided to clinicians on appropriate follow-up for abnormal imaging.

Abbreviations: CT, computed tomography; RCA, root cause analysis.

a trainee, this should be disclosed as well. If the error was caused by a provider not involved in direct patient care, for example, a pharmacist, the primary clinician involved in the patient's care should disclose the error, although that provider should be invited to join. The disclosure should still follow the steps outlined earlier.[32] Of course, great care must be taken to avoid speculation, blaming, or insinuation about other care providers.

OTHER CONSIDERATIONS

Some states have legal protection centered around disclosure and litigation. Many states have adopted "apology laws," which protect some information discussed in disclosures. These laws vary by state, with some protecting only expressions of

---

Box 1
Do's and Don'ts of disclosing medical errors

- Do's
  - State there was an error
  - Apologize
  - Describe the corrective action that will be done
  - Allow time for questions
- Don'ts
  - Use technical language
  - Blame others
  - Speculate about the cause of the error
  - Promise actions that aren't realistic
  - Be defensive

---

sympathy and others protecting admissions of fault. Clinicians should take time to familiarize themselves with their own state's "apology laws."

Committing medical errors is psychologically damaging to providers. The Journal of the American Medical Association reported the results of a focus group from 2003 that physicians "experienced powerful emotions following medical errors and felt upset and guilty about harming the patients. The most difficult challenge was forgiving themselves for the error."[36] Because of this trauma experienced by providers, it is critical that providers feel supported by both their colleagues and institution when an error occurs. Self-forgiveness for committing a medical error is key. Four steps have been identified on the path to self-forgiveness: responsibility, remorse, restoration, and renewal. First, the clinician needs to take responsibility for the error. Second, they should let themselves feel remorse or guilt, thus hopefully mitigating feelings of shame. Next, the clinician must welcome restoration, or try to make amends for the error. Finally, the clinician should allow for renewal or release of negative emotion associated with the error.[36] The lengthy medical training that providers endure does not usually cover this process of self-forgiveness, nor does it cover the expectation that medical errors will occur during their career and the importance of disclosure of medical errors. To improve the rate of medical error disclosures, institutions and medical training programs should be dedicated to supporting those that have committed the error by providing appropriate guidance on both areas of clinical improvement and self-forgiveness.

DISCUSSION

The definitions of medical error described in this article are outcome-driven definitions; that is, the end is used to justify a judgment about the process. There have been proposals to expand its definition to be process dependent. In 1990, Reason defined medical error as a failure of a planned action to be completed as intended (error in execution) or the use of a wrong plan to achieve an aim (error in planning) as well as deviations from the process of care, which may or may not cause harm to the patient.[19] This definition is a departure from the outcome-driven definitions of medical error and is process-driven but fails to look at errors of omission (ie, no plan or action taken) and may be too general in its definition of process of care. Thus, currently, it seems more generally practical to continue to use outcome definitions of medical error: actions either of omission or commission that lead to preventable or ameliorable adverse events, near misses, delays in care or diagnosis, or unanticipated outcomes.

Just as there is debate about a clear definition of medical error, there has been debate about definitions of medical harm. Although there are several harm scales available, there are many difficulties in assessing potential and actual harm, as evidenced by low inter-rater reliability among clinicians in review panels.[37] Thus, some studies suggest engaging 2 or more clinicians as well as evidence-based tools into processes that can achieve better consensus.[38] Furthermore, reviews rely on medical records to determine if potential or actual harm occurred to the patient—and for this method to be valid, the records must contain comprehensive and accurate information.

Despite the complexities and subtleties of defining medical error and harm, it is clear that medical errors significantly impact patients and their families. Medical errors contribute to diminishing trust in the health care system; however, disclosing errors minimizes perceived harm to patients. Error disclosure also serves as an opportunity for improvement through robust collaboration. To rebuild and maintain trust in the health care system, patients should be notified of the error and invited to participate in efforts to identify and prevent future errors. Patients and families are more likely to respond more positively to errors when they receive an acknowledgment of the error, including an explanation of what occurred, expression of remorse, and an explicit apology.[20,30] The broad heterogeneous themes of patients' perceptions of error demonstrate the wide array of differences in needs of patients once an error has occurred.[20] Studies show that the most important factor in people's decisions to file lawsuits is not provider negligence, but ineffective communication between patients and providers.

Malpractice suits often result when an unexpected adverse outcome is met with a lack of empathy from physicians and a perceived or actual withholding of essential information. Often, physicians and other health care professionals have a fear of increased litigation with error disclosure. However, this fear is unfounded: effective disclosure of errors has been shown to reduce legal costs for hospitals, insurers, and providers while also showing increased satisfaction in health care providers from patients.[33] In fact, after the University of Michigan health care system and the VA at Lexington adopted aggressive disclosure programs, they saw a significant decrease in lawsuit numbers and litigation-associated costs.[33]

SUMMARY

Recognition and disclosure of errors are 2 imperative contributions to patient safety culture in health care. Medical errors are common and include adverse events, delays in care, near misses, delays in diagnosis, and unanticipated outcomes. Physical and emotional harm is experienced from medical errors by patients and their families and is classified as potential or actual and graded in severity. Disclosing medical errors and apologizing for the error minimizes perceived harm of error by patients, decreases litigation, and rebuilds trust in the health care system. Future work focused on further improving and normalizing the process if error disclosure is necessary. Disclosure requirements and guidelines on disclosure increase clinician comfort with disclosure while also improving patient acceptance of medical error. Hospitals and medical schools should consider including training on disclosing errors for students, residents, and faculty.

CLINICS CARE POINTS

- If there was a deviation from standard practice that either resulted in harm to the patient or could have resulted in harm to the patient, a medical error occurred.

- Consider using a harm scale to measure harm caused to the patient. The NCC-MERP, HAMEC classification, WHO classification, AHRQ HARM scale, and the American Society of Healthcare and Risk Management (ASHRM) harm scale are examples of validated scales.
- Familiarize yourself with your state's apologies laws to ease some of the anxiety around revealing medical errors.
- If an error has occurred, disclose it to the patient and/or family. First, begin by stating that there has been an error, then describe the course of events using nontechnical language, then state the nature of the mistake, consequence and corrective action, express regret and apologize, elicit questions or concerns, and address them and finally plan the next steps with the patient.
- After an error has occurred, plan a debriefing session with all interested parties and multidisciplinary analysis to prevent future errors. Bringing patients and families into this process, if desired, can be mutually beneficial.
- After the error has been disclosed, recognize that this may be extremely distressing for all parties involved. As the clinician, you should take responsibility for the error, let yourself feel guilt, welcome feelings of restoration, and then finally release negative emotion associated with the error. Seek support from your institution and colleagues to help with this process.

DISCLOSURE

The authors have nothing to disclose.

REFERENCES

1. Makary MA, Daniel M. Medical error-the third leading cause of death in the US. BMJ 2016;353:i2139.
2. Hayward RA, Hofer TP. Estimating hospital deaths due to medical errors: preventability is in the eye of the reviewer. JAMA 2001;286(4):415–20.
3. Gallagher TH, Waterman AD, Ebers AG, et al. Patients' and physicians' attitudes regarding the disclosure of medical errors. JAMA 2003;289(8):1001–7.
4. Moser RH. Diseases of medical progress. N Engl J Med 1956;255(13):606–14.
5. Andel C, Davidow SL, Hollander M, et al. The economics of health care quality and medical errors. J Health Care Finance 2012;39(1):39–50.
6. Brennan TA, Leape LL, Laird NM, et al. Incidence of adverse events and negligence in hospitalized patients: results of the Harvard Medical Practice Study I. 1991. Qual Saf Health Care 2004;13(2):145–51, discussion 151-2.
7. Leape LL, Brennan TA, Laird N, et al. The nature of adverse events in hospitalized patients. Results of the Harvard Medical Practice Study II. N Engl J Med 1991; 324(6):377–84.
8. Thomas EJ, Studdert DM, Burstin HR, et al. Incidence and types of adverse events and negligent care in Utah and Colorado. Med Care 2000;38(3):261–71.
9. Wilson RM, Harrison BT, Gibberd RW, et al. An analysis of the causes of adverse events from the Quality in Australian health care study. Med J Aust 1999;170(9): 411–5.
10. Wilson RM, Runciman WB, Gibberd RW, et al. Quality in Australian health care study. Med J Aust 1996;164(12):754.
11. Grober ED, Bohnen JM. Defining medical error. Can J Surg 2005;48(1):39–44.
12. Friedman SM, Provan D, Moore S, et al. Errors, near misses and adverse events in the emergency department: what can patients tell us? CJEM 2008;10(5):421–7.

13. Reason J, Manstead A, Stradling S, et al. Errors and violations on the roads: a real distinction? Ergonomics 1990;33(10–11):1315–32.
14. Reason JT. Organizational accidents revisited. Second edition. Ashgate; 2015. cm.
15. Hartwig SC, Denger SD, Schneider PJ. Severity-indexed, incident report-based medication error-reporting program. Am J Hosp Pharm 1991;48(12):2611–6.
16. Gates PJ, Baysari MT, Mumford V, et al. Standardising the classification of harm associated with medication errors: the harm associated with medication error classification (HAMEC). Drug Saf 2019;42(8):931–9.
17. Organization WH, ed. Conceptual framework for the internation classification for patient safety. 2009.
18. Williams T, Szekendi M, Pavkovic S, et al. The reliability of AHRQ common format harm scales in rating patient safety events. J Patient Saf 2015;11(1):52–9.
19. Michelle Hoppes JM. Series safety events: a focus on harm classification: deviation in case as link. AMSHRM white paper series 2012;2 (1):1-32.
20. Kathleen M, Mazor SLG, Dodd K, Alper Eric. Understanding patients' perceptions of medical errors. J Community Health 2013;2(1):34–6.
21. Northcott H, Vanderheyden L, Northcott J, et al. Perceptions of preventable medical errors in Alberta, Canada. Int J Qual Health Care 2008;20(2):115–22.
22. blendon RJ, DesRoches CM, Brodie M, et al. Views of practicing physicians and the public on medical errors. N Engl J Med 2002;347(24):1933–40.
23. Hickson Gerald BEWC, Bithens Penny G, Sloan Frank A. Factors that prompted families to file medical malpractice claims following perinatal injuries. JAMA 1992; 267:1359–63.
24. Levinson W, Roter DL, Mullooly JP, et al. Physician-patient communication. the relationship with malpractice claims among primary care physicians and surgeons. JAMA 1997;277(7):553–9.
25. Vincent C. Understanding and responding to adverse events. N Engl J Med 2003;348(11):1051–6.
26. christine duclos me, taylor leslie, quintela javan. debora main, wilson pace and elizabeth staton. Patient persepctive of patient-provider communcation after adverse events. Int J Qual Health Care 2005;17(6):479–86.
27. Koeck DSaCM. What makes an error unaccepatble? a factorial survey on the disclosure of medical errors. Intern Int J Qual Health Care 2004;16(4):317–26.
28. Wolf ZR, Hughes RG. Error reporting and disclosure. In: Hughes RG, editor. Patient safety and quality: an evidence-based handbook for nurses. 2008. *Advances in Patient Safety.*
29. Forum NQ. Safe practices for better healthcare. Am J Health-Syst Pharm 2009; 66(8):702.
30. Mazor KM, Simon SR, Yood RA, et al. Health plan members' views about disclosure of medical errors. Ann Intern Med 2004;140(6):409–18.
31. Levinson W, Yeung J, Ginsburg S. Disclosure of medical error. JAMA 2016; 316(7):764–5.
32. Gallagher TH, Mello MM, Levinson W, et al. Talking with patients about other clinicians' errors. N Engl J Med 2013;369(18):1752–7.
33. Clinton HR, Obama B. Making patient safety the centerpiece of medical liability reform. N Engl J Med 2006;354(21):2205–8.
34. Gallagher TH, Studdert D, Levinson W. Disclosing harmful medical errors to patients. N Engl J Med 2007;356(26):2713–9.
35. Berthold j. Disclosing medical errors the right way. Internal Medicine; 2014.

36. Berlinger N. Resolving harmful medical mistakes-is there a role for forgiveness? Virtual Mentor 2011;13(9):647–54.
37. Forrey RA, Pedersen CA, Schneider PJ. Interrater agreement with a standard scheme for classifying medication errors. Am J Health Syst Pharm 2007;64(2): 175–81.
38. Morimoto T, Gandhi TK, Seger AC, et al. Adverse drug events and medication errors: detection and classification methods. Qual Saf Health Care 2004;13(4): 306–14.

When Communication Breaks Down

Handling Hostile Patients

Martha Ward, MD[a,b],*, Sarah Cook, MD[a]

KEYWORDS

- Hostility • Anger • Therapeutic alliance • Communication • Countertransference
- Active listening

KEY POINTS

- Difficult patient encounters are common, and many involve patient hostility.
- Patient hostility generally occurs from broken communication and/or a mismatch in goals in the patient-physician dyad.
- Specific patient, physician, and situational factors can contribute to patient hostility, and such factors should be identified and addressed.
- Healing the breach in the health care alliance requires inquiry into the cause of the patient's anger, active listening, collaboration on next steps, and patient empowerment in creating a common goal.

INTRODUCTION

Nearly every physician has experienced it: the heartsink feeling of approaching a patient encounter anticipated as being difficult. It may occur when viewing a particular patient's name on the clinic schedule or when gearing up to enter the room of a disgruntled inpatient. Challenging patient encounters are fairly common; in fact, up to 15% of patient-physician encounters are deemed "difficult" by physicians.[1]

Although there are a number of potential reasons for difficult interactions with patients, many of these encounters result from a breakdown of communication and a breach in the health care alliance, overtly manifest as patient hostility. Such care breaches are challenging for both doctor and patient and can lead to many adverse outcomes. Difficult patient encounters significantly contribute to low job satisfaction and physician burnout.[2] After a challenging patient encounter, physicians report significant frustration and unease and admit to secretly hoping that the "difficult" patient

[a] Department of Psychiatry and Behavioral Sciences, Emory University School of Medicine, 100 Woodruff Circle, Atlanta, GA 30322; [b] Department of Medicine, Emory University School of Medicine, 100 Woodruff Circle, Atlanta, GA 30322.
* Corresponding author. 100 Woodruff Circle, Atlanta, GA 30322.
E-mail address: mcraig@emory.edu

Med Clin N Am 106 (2022) 689–703
https://doi.org/10.1016/j.mcna.2022.01.009
0025-7125/22/© 2022 Elsevier Inc. All rights reserved.

would not return for follow-up.[3] Patients likewise suffer from such interactions, which result in costly care-seeking, lack of trust in the medical system, incomplete or poor patient care, and worse medical outcomes.[4]

Studies and literature on "difficult patients" have identified some patient factors that lead to bad interactions and patient hostility, and increasingly it is recognized that physician and situational factors contribute. In this article, the authors focus on the various factors that may lead to patient hostility, with suggestions for how to approach such situations in order to prevent or heal breaches in the health care alliance.

CURRENT EVIDENCE
Patient Characteristics: Psychiatric Diagnoses

Specific inherent patient characteristics can predispose individuals to hostile engagement with the medical system. Included among these are various psychiatric diagnoses, including personality disorders, mood disorders, anxiety disorders, and substance use disorders (**Table 1**).

Personality disorders

Personality disorders consist of an enduring pattern of inner experience and behavior that differs markedly from cultural norms and includes alterations in ways of perceiving self and others, appropriate affective range and intensity, interpersonal relationships, and controlling impulses.[4,5] The very nature of such disorders imbues fragility in times of stress and an inflexibility in coping with adversity, a clear setup for challenges with medical illness. In addition to the internal turmoil experienced by those with personality disorders, affected patients also tend to disrupt the environment around them. Such patients may display hostility toward the treatment team and mistrust of treatments offered. They may show extremes of emotion with rapid escalation when they perceive that their needs are not being met, particularly when fearing abandonment at hospital discharge. They may make frequent demands, with particular preferences for their care that seem illogical. They may "split" their preferences for team members, identifying clear favorites and enemies. Because of these behaviors, patients with personality disorders, particularly borderline personality disorder, often evoke strong emotional reactions in the care team.[4]

Although personality disorders are likely highly prevalent (research suggests that 1 in 4 patients in primary care meet criteria), they can be challenging to diagnose because of overlapping characteristics between the different personality disorders and other mental illnesses. Referral to a psychiatrist, if the patient is amenable, can help with diagnostic clarification, psychotherapeutic intervention, and potential pharmacotherapy. For the nonpsychiatrist physician, there are several interventions that can help to address hostile behaviors that disrupt treatment, including communication strategies to engage in the moment to diffuse patient hostility (**Table 2**). It can be helpful to check the team's emotions, recognize the emotional toll that the patient may be placing on certain members, and offer support to the patient. Individuals with personality disorders are often raised in invalidating environments and fear rejection and abandonment; acknowledging and naming emotions can be validating. Establishing boundaries with consistent rules regarding appointments or how quickly the patient's calls will be returned can help to create a neutral environment in which erratic help-seeking is not rewarded. Often, such patients have received attention only with escalation of emotion, reinforcing their lability. Physicians can alter this pattern by reinforcing desired behaviors (eg, calm interactions) by increasing attention and, when appropriate, removing engagement when the patient is acting out: "You seem upset. I don't think we are going to be able to work on this problem right now." Care team

Table 1
Patient factors contributing to patient hostility

Patient Characteristic	Clinical Difficulty	Physician's Coping Strategies
Psychiatric diagnoses		
Personality disorders	Fragility in times of stress Mistrust of treatment team Rapid escalation of emotion Frequent demands Splitting	Psychiatric referral Recognize emotions in treatment team; offer support Name emotions Establish boundaries/rules Reinforce desired behaviors and extinguish acting-out behaviors Encourage self-efficacy
Mood/anxiety disorder	Somatic complaints Diagnostic difficulty Poor adherence Help-seeking/rejecting	Screen and treat Address stigma Referral to psychiatric/psychological services as needed
Substance use disorder	Defensive when asked about use Concern for manipulation	Use motivational interviewing Check biases Use neutral external agreements
Medical diagnoses		
Chronic pain	Unrealistic expectations Undisclosed underlying fears Anger at undertreatment Physician hypervigilance in the era of the opioid epidemic	Create reasonable, clear expectations Set goals related to function Check biases Screen for comorbid psychiatric disorders Offer psychological support Refer to multidisciplinary pain management
Somatic symptom disorders	Patient distress out of proportion to physical illness Frustration with treatment Help-seeking/rejecting Fear of "missing something" Unfounded referrals and testing	Use rational medical decision making Validate symptom severity Reassure patient regarding ruled out diagnoses Inquire into meaning for patient Screen for trauma Schedule regular visits Focus on symptom control rather than cure

(continued on next page)

		Physician's Coping
Table 1 (*continued*)		
Patient Characteristic	**Clinical Difficulty**	**Strategies**
Behaviors and beliefs		
"Demanding" patient	Mismatch in patient/doctor goals Patient requests nonindicated, expensive, or harmful treatments and tests Patient believes doctor is withholding	Reassure patient of ethical obligation to give optimal treatment Explain reasoning Maintain integrity of practice
"Self-destructive saboteur"	Treatment nonadherence Poor self-care Physician questions efficacy Psychosocial challenges	Expose hidden curriculum of "good" and "bad" patient Address social determinants of health Celebrate small successes Set realistic goals Embrace "good enough"
Patient biases	Physician hurt, anger, and harm Breakdown in therapeutic alliance Worse patient outcomes Impaired workflow	Triage patient care according to acuity and decision making Establish institutional policy Support targets of bias

members can also validate while encouraging self-efficacy: "I see you are angry right now. What usually helps you in these situations?"[4]

Mood and anxiety disorders

A wide body of literature supports the association of depressive and anxiety disorders with difficult patient-doctor encounters.[1] Furthermore, patients with certain disorders, such as obstructive sleep apnea, experience psychological distress, which has been linked to high levels of hostility.[6] Patients who have unrecognized mood and anxiety disorders may present with multiple somatic complaints that do not respond to targeted treatments. Such complaints may shift focus and present diagnostic difficulty, frustrating both patient and physician alike. Lack of treatment efficacy leads to poor adherence and mistrust of the physician and their ability, with patients in cycles of help-seeking/rejecting.[7] In order to optimally avoid patient hostility in such cases, underlying mood and anxiety disorders must be screened for, recognized, diagnosed, and treated. Successfully addressing such illnesses may require greater understanding of cultural barriers and a discussion regarding stigma. Treatment may be successfully initiated by a nonpsychiatrist physician using selective serotonin reuptake inhibitors or another first-line antidepressant, at an appropriate dose and duration. Formal psychological support with a trained therapist or psychiatrist may also be initiated if patient preference and resources allow.

Substance use disorders

Patients with substance use disorders exhibit loss of control and continued use despite physical, emotional, and/or social consequences. Hostility may arise when

Table 2
Communication strategies to redirect patient hostility[1]

Strategy	Physician Action	Examples
Active listening	Allow patient to talk without interruption Allow silence Use facilitation and interpretation to encourage disclosure Use body language to display nonjudgmental attention (eye contact, open stance)	"I heard that you felt disrespected. Can you tell me more about that?" "Please help me to understand the issues that are important here." "Can you help me understand why you are upset?"
Validate and empathize	Name the emotion Agree with the emotion if possible	"I can see you are angry." "It sounds like this diagnosis is scary." "I can understand why you would be upset about having to wait so long."
Explore solutions	Engage the patient in a collaborative manner, using "we" and "us" Allow the patient to regain control of the situation	"How would you like to see this go in the future?" "What ways can we work on this together?" "What else do I need to know to help us better solve this problem?"
Provide closure	Determine a plan that is mutually agreed upon	"What I understand is that next time I'm running late, you'd prefer to reschedule." "What I hear is that you'd prefer to work together to set the agenda for our next meeting, so that your concerns are better addressed."

Cannarella Lorenzetti R, Jacques CH, Donovan C, Cottrell S, Buck J. Managing difficult encounters: understanding physician, patient, and situational factors. *Am Fam Physician*. Mar 15 2013;87(6):419-25.

such patients are queried by the physician about their use, resulting in patient anger and confrontation. In such instances, a patient-centered and nonjudgmental approach should be taken. Motivational interviewing is an evidence-based technique for addressing patient ambivalence regarding adverse health behaviors and has been shown to have efficacy in many disorders, including substance use. The use of motivational interviewing allows the patient and physician to explore the patient's desire, need, ability, and reason for making a change.[7] In addition, patients with substance use disorders may become hostile when physicians fail to prescribe a substance of misuse, such as opioids or benzodiazepines. This becomes particularly challenging when patients have an indicated reason for taking the medication. Physicians must be vigilant to check their own biases and not automatically label patients as "drug-seeking," particularly if physical dependence requires higher doses to successfully treat a condition ("pseudo addiction"). Pain medication contracts and vigilant use of state patient drug monitoring programs help to introduce neutrality and avoid negotiation. However, when manipulation, misuse, and diversion are occurring, physicians must understand that there is an essential mismatch in the patient and physician goal and realize that the patient may not be satisfied with the interaction.

Patient Characteristics: Medical Diagnoses

In addition to psychiatric illnesses, several medical syndromes have been associated with challenging clinical encounters and have the potential to induce patient hostility. Most frequently cited among these are patients suffering from chronic pain and those with somatic or functional syndromes.

Chronic pain

Individuals who suffer from chronic pain may display anger for many reasons. They may have unrealistic treatment hopes and expectations; often pain can be reduced in intensity but not removed. They may have fears about the meaning of their pain, and concern for undiagnosed causes. They may be undertreated for their pain because of the provider's unconscious bias; it has been repeatedly demonstrated that African Americans suffer undertreatment of pain in the hospital setting.[8] They may have the experience of being labeled as "drug-seeking." Supposed "red flags" that alert the physician to "drug-seeking" behavior include many behaviors that are common for individuals with recurrent pain crises, such as those with sickle cell disease: citing the dose and name of a preferred analgesic, preferring injections to oral medications, and instructing the nurse where and at what rate to administer the analgesic.[8] Hypervigilance concerning "drug-seeking" has blossomed in the era of the opioid epidemic, with skepticism about the efficacy of opioids for noncancer pain resulting in regulations and practice parameters.[8]

Physicians can more effectively treat their patients with chronic pain by using several strategies. First, set up expectations early: "your pain will probably not go away completely, but each thing we do has the potential to improve it." Engage patients in goal-setting that relates to function rather than pain intensity. Set up small, discrete, proximal goals as well as long-term goals. As discussed previously, check biases regarding "drug-seeking" and rule out "pseudo addiction." Finally, address the emotional component of pain, screening for depression or anxiety disorders, or a history of trauma and posttraumatic stress disorder. Offer psychological support if available, even if a formal psychiatric diagnosis is not made. If possible, refer patients to a formal multidisciplinary pain management team.[7,9]

Somatic symptom disorders

Somatic symptom disorders consist of a broad range of presenting complaints and are defined as distressing somatic symptoms that are accompanied by abnormal thoughts, feelings, or behaviors in response to these symptoms. The diagnosis does not indicate the absence of a medical basis for illness, but instead highlights the elevated level of distress experienced by patients who suffer from these disorders.[10] As discussed in the previous section on anxiety and depression, unexplained somatic symptoms can lead to frustration, care-seeking/rejecting behavior, and lack of trust in the medical system. For physicians, these can present a diagnostic dilemma and a treatment challenge, with fears that an underlying diagnosis may be missed, resulting in extensive testing and referrals. Physicians should focus on rational medical decision making, following best practice guidelines whenever possible to avoid unnecessary referrals and diagnostic testing. In discussions with the patient, it is essential to validate symptom severity while reassuring the patient that the worst diagnoses have been ruled out via before testing. Inquiries surrounding the emotional/psychological meaning of the symptoms should be posed: "What do you think may be causing this? Have you known anyone else with these symptoms? What was their outcome?" Providing time for the patient to offer their thoughts about their symptoms allows integration of their physical symptoms with emotional experience, a key component of healing. Emotional integration allows the patient to feel understood and supported and therefore encourages emotional and physical relief. Inquiring about the patient's experience also gives greater context for both the patient and the physician. Screening for trauma and abuse may also uncover a psychological cause of physical pain. Regular outpatient visits should be scheduled, to provide reassurance and to avoid emergency visits, and to assess any new or changing symptoms in a rational manner.[11] Finally, it may be beneficial to reformulate the treatment plan to focus on alleviating symptoms rather than curing the condition.[1,7]

Patient Characteristics: Behaviors and Beliefs

Finally, patients may display certain behaviors that foster an oppositional relationship between patient and physician. These include patients who are labeled as demanding or nonadherent or who display bias against the social identity of the physician.

The "demanding" patient

As discussed previously regarding patients with substance use disorders, conflict can easily arise when the goal of the patient and the physician is not in accord. In the age of the Internet, information is readily available to patients. Information gleaned may be unreliable, may be interpreted incorrectly, or may build fear of the presence of an unlikely but catastrophic diagnosis. Based on this information, patients may request medications or diagnostic testing that is not indicated, costly, or harmful. Patients may react with anger if they assess that the physician is withholding a necessary medication or test. In such cases, it is essential for the physician to reassure the patient that they would honor the request if it were in the patient's best interest, and to be transparent with reasoning regarding risks, benefits, and current best practices. Unfortunately, it may be necessary to realize that some patients may leave the encounter angry, as that is the cost of maintaining integrity in the practice of medicine.[7]

"Self-destructive saboteur"

Treatment nonadherence and poor self-care are associated with high levels of patient hostility,[12] likely mediated by poor social support networks, low socioeconomic status, and low levels of education.[12,13] Physician reactions to nonadherence to treatment recommendations fuel the fire of patient hostility. Although some of the frustration that physicians express is conscious and overt, the unconscious impression of the "bad," "noncompliant" patient is indoctrinated early in medical training.[14] Patients seen as "good" possess cultural health capital: language facility, proactive attitude toward knowledge accumulation, and application of such knowledge to the biomedical approach to disease management. Those with cultural health capital receive greater care and attention, more empathy, and more respect. "Bad" patients, with lower health literacy and capital, are considered guilty of causing or perpetrating their illness.[14] The internalization of this model enforces inequality based on class and often race. Rectifying this model requires disrupting the hidden curriculum of medical training, where patients are labeled as "bad" or "good," and improving the ability of physicians to recognize and act on unconscious bias. On an individual level, physicians can improve patient-doctor dynamics regarding treatment adherence by addressing psychosocial reasons for nonadherence, including access and health literacy. Physicians can also work with patients to celebrate small successes and set realistic goals, embracing the idea of "good enough."[1,7]

Patient biases

Physician social identity characteristics—race, ethnicity, sex, disability, gender presentation, sexual orientation—may be the target of demeaning and hostile patient language or behavior. Unfortunately, this phenomenon is not uncommon, with 59% of physicians reporting identity-based patient bias in one survey.[15] Such interactions harm both patients and physicians, resulting in harm in those targeted, breakdown in the therapeutic alliance, worse patient health outcomes, and impaired workflow at the expense of other patients.[16] Often such patients request physician reassignment, a conundrum which must consider patient interests, medical personnel employment rights, and the duty to treat. A treatment algorithm based on patient acuity and decision-making capacity has been proposed by Paul-Emile and colleagues.[17] Institutional policies are necessary given the increasing diversification of the health care workforce. Such policies should include consideration for various provider roles (nurses, trainees), a reporting structure, support for recipients of bias, as well as mechanisms and training for addressing bias.[15] The cumulative impact of such aggressions on the health care provider cannot be overestimated. Acknowledgment, discussion, upstanding, and support are essential.

Physician Characteristics

Patient hostility results from a discordance in the physician-patient dyad, with an incongruity among traits, needs, and behaviors. Although several studies have clarified patient factors associated with difficult interactions, there is a relative dearth of data on physician factors that may instigate patient hostility. Some of the quantified physician characteristics associated with difficult patient interactions include age, gender, attitude toward psychosocial aspects of patient care, stress and hours worked, and psychiatric diagnosis in the physician.

Age/gender

Although data are mixed, there is limited evidence that younger age is associated with higher prevalence of difficult patient interactions.[2,18] Several factors may contribute to this, including inexperience and lower confidence in provider ability. Physicians trained in an era of metrics aimed at patient satisfaction may have internalized a less-robust sense of agency than those steeped in the paternalism of old. In addition, female gender has been variably associated with greater difficulty in patient interaction.[18] This may be attributed to the higher incidence of neuroticism in women[19]; neuroticism has been associated with higher rates of adverse emotional states, such as anger, guilt, and frustration. Perhaps more tangible are the gender differences in structural context in the lives of women versus men (family responsibility, child-rearing).[13] Although age and gender are not intervenable characteristics, the associated factors that bring challenges in patient care should be addressed. Improving self-efficacy, combating imposter syndrome, and sharing of family responsibilities would all go a long way to alleviating the burden that young women face in pursuing careers in medicine.

Discomfort with addressing psychosocial health

In a recent study of 500 outpatient visits, the strongest predictor of a "difficult" encounter was physician discomfort with addressing aspects of psychosocial health.[3] This finding is consistent with previous studies documenting lower patient and physician satisfaction with communication styles that favored a narrowly "biomedical" focus.[20] Patients internalized by physicians as "bad" and displaying greater hostility suffer from a higher burden of adverse social determinants of health, such as those associated with poverty.[14] It is increasingly clear that the context of the patient in community and society is an essential part of care, and greater facility with addressing these elements of a patient's life is a critical skill for physicians.

Stress and psychiatric diagnosis

It is not surprising that physicians with high stress ratings, and those that report high levels of fatigue and burnout, experience more challenging patient encounters. In one study, physicians in the highest category of rating patients as difficult were 12.2 times more likely to be burned out than those in the lowest category of rating patients as difficult.[18] Overwork contributes to physician stress and difficulty relating to patients. Physicians who work greater than 55 hours per week are statistically more likely to experience difficult patient encounters than those who work less.[18] Finally, psychiatric diagnoses in the physician, such as depression and anxiety, are associated with challenging patient encounters.[18] Appropriate attention and care for the psychological distress of the health care team are essential to improving patient affective states and outcomes.

Less quantifiable physician characteristics

In addition to these studied physician traits, less quantifiable physician characteristics likely play an important role in the physician-patient dyad. These include countertransference, physician personality traits, and personal expectations of the physician.

Countertransference

Countertransference plays a prominent yet often unacknowledged role in medical relationships (**Box 1**). Even within psychiatry, countertransference is often not well explained to medical students, residents, or practicing physicians. Although physicians frequently learn of transference, countertransference, or the physician's unconscious and conscious feelings toward a patient, is seldom discussed.[21] Reasons for lack of discussion include limited opportunities and fear of self-disclosure of perceived personal failings, family history, or trauma. Physicians may struggle with revealing personal aspects of their lives, such as family dynamics or challenging experiences in childhood, which are often 2 major aspects contributing to countertransference. In addition, training physicians must navigate the art of maintaining professional relationships and may not have appropriate avenues available to disclose private aspects of their lives in a constructive way. Unfortunately, an understanding and ability to address countertransference are key because they exist with every patient to varying degrees and are almost certainly at play during difficult patient encounters.

Over time, the term countertransference has focused more on the interaction between both patient and physician characteristics rather than simply the physician's history or personality traits. Winnicott describes how clinicians frequently react to patients in the same ways as other people in the patient's life do, and therefore, countertransference reveals useful information about the patient's life and relationships. Thus, countertransference is viewed as a jointly created phenomenon with contributing factors from both the physician and the patient[21] rather than only the physician's personal attributes.[22] Countertransference at work is most clearly seen in projective identification, when aspects of the patient's intrapsychic world are projected onto the physician, and the physician's subjective experience of this is influenced by history and personality. Although usually the feelings aroused in the physician during projective identification are uncomfortable, countertransference enactments can be opportunities for growth and containment in the therapeutic relationship.

Personality traits

Medical education has long valued, and in many programs has favored other characteristics, certain personality traits, namely confidence, emotional toughness, and assertiveness.[23] In a study on physician personalities using the Five Factor Model, physicians, residents, and medical students scored highly for conscientiousness compared with the general public.[24] Conscientiousness in the Five Factor Model is defined as efficient, organized, planning, reliable, responsible, and thorough. With such a strong focus on these characteristics, a physician's expression of emotional difficulties with a patient became uncomfortable to discuss, if not taboo. Affect neutrality often becomes the silent rule, so encounters with "difficult patients" become even more challenging, as physicians suppress their feelings, and patient classifications and stereotypes about the challenging patient become more entrenched.[14] In addition, throughout their education and training, physicians are encouraged to follow rules and uphold the medical hierarchy. Physicians who are organized and less flexible succeeded more frequently in traditional medical settings, and individuals attracted to medicine include those who appreciate control and mastery of academics. Many physicians are "people pleasers" and may thrive on praise from others, particularly supervisors or patients to whom they provide a service. Satisfactory interactions with patients that evoke positive emotions validate physicians' desire to please and the time and energy poured into study and training. Successful physicians are frequently described as having a strong work ethic, and the years of education and training are highlighted when patients look for a "good doctor."

It is not surprising, therefore, that physician factors, when viewed in the context of difficult patient encounters, contribute to a perfect storm. Whereas physicians are conscientious, difficult patients are stereotyped as not having control over their health or behaviors and are not perceived to "follow the rules," such as taking medications as prescribed or following up consistently. Physicians, when working with a patient where the treatment plan is not proceeding as planned, or the medical interaction feels fraught, might view a challenging patient as disorganized and uninterested in participating in their care on one hand, or demanding and ungrateful on the other hand. Difficult patient interactions prevent physicians from feeling satisfied in their work and challenge the idea that their years of education and training culminated in success. Clearly, the discord between typical physician characteristics and perceived difficult patient qualities and behaviors sets up a challenging dynamic.

Box 1
Understanding Countertransference

A simple example of countertransference is as follows:

A physician with a family member who suffered from alcohol use disorder during the physician's early childhood feels increasingly frustrated, anxious, and irritated with a patient who has a substance use disorder. There has not been any significant event or challenging interaction, but the physician dreads appointments with this patient without knowing why and finds herself treating the patient harshly compared with her other patients. She feels emotionally drained after interacting with this patient despite a pleasant, routine visit without complicating factors. The physician meets with a therapist and, while describing her upset with the patient, remembers neglect from the family member with alcohol use disorder she experienced at the age of four. She recalls feeling overwhelmed and scared by having to care for this person when they were intoxicated.

Personal expectations

Similarly, many physicians enter the medical field with specific expectations that can play a role in difficult moments with patients. Some physicians entered the field with more entrenched traditional views about medicine, including a conscious or unconscious expectation of holding power. Physicians are historically revered as knowledgeable, well-respected leaders, and many physicians enter the field expecting their interactions with patients to reflect this ideal. In contrast, changes in the medical system, including decreased time available for patient care and less control over treatment options, impact the physician reputation and freedom in their practice, impacting their reputation with patients, particularly those with more challenging needs. When treating patients during a challenging interaction, the physician's expectations of their role as a well-respected leader with power can drastically change.

The realization during difficult patient encounters that a physician may not be as powerful or respected as expected impacts another physician expectation: pride. Physicians spend years of time studying and training, often giving up special moments with family and friends as well as time for their own personal development. When engaged with a patient in a challenging dynamic, physicians' sense of pride may be threatened and could certainly exacerbate or fuel a difficult interaction.

Finally, when considering personal expectations of the physician, it is likely that nearly every physician entering the field does so with the goal of helping others in some way, whether from extending or improving quality of life to simply being a caring presence in the patient's life. Altruistic motivation helps physicians continue a daunting, rigorous education and training course, and for most physicians, drives career satisfaction and impacts longevity of practice. A physician's altruistic goals are directly confronted during challenging patient encounters; some of the most difficult experiences a physician has working with patients are usually when a patient asserts that a physician is not helping them, or, even worse, is causing the patient suffering. These experiences cause surprise and hurt for the medical student, resident, or new or well-established physician, who must come to terms with the idea that the patient's perception of them during an uncomfortable moment contrasts with their expectations.

APPROACH
Addressing Nonquantifiable Physician Characteristics

Countertransferential reactions, individual personality characteristics, and physician expectations are generally less overt and thus may be challenging to successfully address. As an initial step, self-reflection may bring forth a greater understanding of how the physician's thoughts, feelings, and behaviors are contributing to patient hostility. Research supports this action: physicians who are aware of and accept their emotions may have better emotional intelligence and thus better patient-doctor relationships.[25] Physicians may begin by identifying patients that they perceive as difficult, by recognizing the onset of a "heartsink" feeling, or pinpointing the patients that they most often avoid or make the focus of humor. Once such patients are identified, physicians may obtain valuable clues to the nature of the difficulty by carefully observing their emotional response that the patient elicits. Improved physician insight and appreciation for patient experience may also be achieved through the regular practice of mindfulness or appreciative inquiry.[26,27]

Discussion of difficult patient interactions with others can also provide perspective and insight. Balint groups were first created in the 1950s as a weekly discussion group for general practitioners in London to review case histories of patients. These have evolved to focus on the aspects of physicians' personalities and emotions that contribute to challenging patient encounters, and often exist as a mandatory part of training in the field of psychiatry.[11] Such groups increase empathy in medical students and likely have a similar effect on practicing physicians.[28] Understanding of personal life experiences and their impact on patient interactions may also be achieved through individual psychotherapy.[7]

Finally, when the physician's emotions or actions are continually engendering hostility in the patient, an ethics consult can be of great assistance. Mediation by a third party can be the key to successful negotiation, by allowing the creation of the "third story": an impartial telling of the events that both parties can agree on. Ethics consultation services generally agree that this is in the bandwidth of their practice; in fact, 77% of US ethics consultation services most frequently cited that "resolving real or imagined conflicts" was a central mission of the service.[29]

Addressing Situational Factors

In addition to specific patient and physician characteristics, certain situational or environmental factors can lead to patient anger. Although some of these are unavoidable, steps can be taken to improve patient communication surrounding the circumstance in order to prevent or diffuse hostility. For instance, engage with other care team members, such as the inpatient unit manager or social worker.

Addressing Time Factors

With ever-increasing workloads and the medical complexity of an aging population, time is often short in clinical situations. Often, pathophysiological processes take precedence over the psychological aspects of personhood, making patients feel belittled and rushed.[30] Physicians can impact this by ensuring that they sit down when entering a room, make eye contact while conversing, and ask at least one general question about the individual's well-being or personal life.[1] If the patient suffers from multimorbidity, the physician may plan for longer or more frequent visits, or schedule the visit at the start or the end of the day.[1] Running late is often inevitable and is a common source of patient hostility. In such cases, an apology and a brief honest explanation can go a long way to healing the rift.[31]

Addressing Language Barriers

In a country with an increasingly diverse population, patients with a primary language other than English are more and more common. Frustration can arise from misunderstandings owing to inept translation or attempts to communicate in partially understood English. Whenever possible, physicians should work with a trained medical interpreter who translates exactly what is said rather than summarizes or edits. This may be optimized by giving short phrases at a time. Physicians should maintain eye contact with the patient while speaking, rather than with the interpreter. Clashes in cultural norms can also create patient unease, particularly if a physician inadvertently offends with speech or behavior. Although global cultural competency is not realistic, physicians should aim to be culturally humble and open to cues from patients.[1]

Addressing Multiple People

Up to 16% of adult outpatient visits include a companion to the primary patient.[32] This has the potential to create a triangulation of interaction, with negative dynamics between the patient and companion, or the companion and the physician. Overly assertive companions may interrupt the physician-patient conversation, causing frustration and resentment. It is essential to determine the reason for the companion's presence: perhaps cultural reasons, or maybe the companion needs to be involved in health care decisions due to the patient's cognitive impairment? Furthermore, is the companion wanted or unwanted? In such circumstances, the physician should spend at least some of the visit with the patient alone to determine if the companion's presence is desired, and for what portion of the visit.[1] If a group of people is involved in the care of a patient, such as in cases where the patient is unable to speak for themselves, a single person should be appointed as the family representative in order to prevent mixed messages or excessive time in discussion.[11]

Addressing the Inpatient Environment

Many aspects of the inpatient environment can invoke patient hostility. Medical interventions, such as NPO orders before a procedure, can seem unwarranted and unnecessary. Although nightly blood draws will not likely ever be welcomed, communicating reasons for diagnostic testing and allowing time for patient questions may help allay anger. Many additional factors can contribute to a sense of loss of control for the patient, leading to anxiety and anger. Every attempt should be made to respect privacy and create as calm of an environment as possible. When possible, physicians should close doors or curtains for conversations. Physicians should ask permission before altering the patient's room environment (eg, turning on the light, turning off the television) or when moving the patient's gown for physical examination. Fragmentation of care, with frequently changing attending physicians, can also negatively impact patient behavior. Physicians must be vigilant to ensure successful transitions of care through excellent sign-out communications and to be sure to introduce themselves when beginning inpatient service.[33]

DISCUSSION

Interactions between physicians and patients, like any interpersonal experience, have the potential to be challenging. Physicians and patients must manage their own characteristics, personal histories, medical complexities, and social and economic concerns, while forging a relationship with one another—a daunting task. Physicians have a unique opportunity to use their medical knowledge and communication skills to collaborate with even the most challenging of patient circumstances, with the understanding that it is natural to have fraught encounters from time to time. Although the difficult interaction may be unavoidable, the opportunity to repair the physician-patient alliance exists and provides relief, and at the very least, understanding the factors involved can help reduce discomfort and stress.

SUMMARY

Although patient hostility may arise from specific characteristics of the patient, physician, or situation, the fracture of the physician-patient dyad generally comes from a mismatch in expectations and a breakdown of communication. The first step in healing the breach is understanding the reason for patient anger, whether overt or unconscious, and taking steps to address such anger. Physicians must recognize that hostility may represent anxiety or a desire to maintain autonomy. It is essential to address and name specific emotions: "I see that you are angry" or "It seems like you are telling me that you're scared." When recognized, anger may be directed at the appropriate entity, such as the disease or the system. Physicians must ally with the patient, reinforcing that the patient is entitled to excellent care and that the physician is on their side. Finally, when the breach in the therapeutic alliance is severe, physicians may want to bring in other members of the health care team to assist, such as ethics consultation teams.

CLINICS CARE POINTS

- Recognize that patient hostility generally arises from a breakdown in communication and can result in a breach in the therapeutic alliance.
- Explore the source of a patient's anger. Anger may be a manifestation of fear, grief, or discontent with prior experiences in the health care system, but there may also be contributions from specific patient, physician, or situational factors.
- Actively listen when inquiring about the patient's hostility.
- To promote self-efficacy and help prevent anger, use collaborative plans to heal breaches in the alliance and empower patients to contribute to their care plan.
- Assess your own emotional responses to patients and seek to understand how your own experiences, personality traits, and biases affect patient interactions.
- Self-reflection and discussion through Balint groups or personal psychotherapy may aid physicians in creating empathy, compassion, and better patient care.
- When the health care breach is serious, consider a second opinion from another colleague, subspecialist, or ethics consultation to create the "third story" from a neutral point of view.

DISCLOSURE

The authors have no financial or commercial conflicts of interest to disclose.

REFERENCES

1. Hull SK, Broquet K. How to manage difficult patient encounters. Fam Pract Manag 2007;14(6):30–4.
2. An PG, Rabatin JS, Manwell LB, et al. Burden of difficult encounters in primary care: data from the minimizing error, maximizing outcomes study. Arch Intern Med 2009;169(4):410–4.
3. Jackson JL, Kroenke K. Difficult patient encounters in the ambulatory clinic: clinical predictors and outcomes. Arch Intern Med 1999;159(10):1069–75.
4. Riddle M, Meeks T, Alvarez C, et al. When personality is the problem: managing patients with difficult personalities on the acute care unit. J Hosp Med 2016; 11(12):873–8.
5. Personality disorders. Diagnostic and Statistical Manual of Mental Disorders.
6. Timkova V, Nagyova I, Reijneveld SA, et al. Psychological distress in patients with obstructive sleep apnoea: the role of hostility and coping self-efficacy. J Health Psychol 2020;25(13–14):2244–59.
7. Cannarella Lorenzetti R, Jacques CH, Donovan C, et al. Managing difficult encounters: understanding physician, patient, and situational factors. Am Fam Physician 2013;87(6):419–25.
8. Rich BA. Distinguishing difficult patients from difficult maladies. Am J Bioeth 2013;13(4):24–6.
9. Gatchel RJ, McGeary DD, McGeary CA, et al. Interdisciplinary chronic pain management: past, present, and future. Am Psychol 2014;69(2):119–30.
10. Kurlansik SL, Maffei MS. Somatic symptom disorder. Am Fam Physician 2016; 93(1):49–54.
11. Breen KJ, Greenberg PB. Difficult physician-patient encounters. Intern Med J 2010;40(10):682–8.
12. Keith F, Krantz DS, Chen R, et al. Anger, hostility, and hospitalizations in patients with heart failure. Health Psychol 2017;36(9):829–38.

13. Tzitzikos G, Kotrotsiou E, Bonotis K, et al. Assessing hostility in patients with chronic obstructive pulmonary disease (COPD). Psychol Health Med 2019; 24(5):605–19.

14. Sointu E. 'Good' patient/'bad' patient: clinical learning and the entrenching of inequality. Sociol Health Illn 2017;39(1):63–77.

15. Paul-Emile K, Critchfield JM, Wheeler M, et al. Addressing patient bias toward health care workers: recommendations for medical centers. Ann Intern Med 2020;173(6):468–73.

16. Singh K, Sivasubramaniam P, Ghuman S, et al. The dilemma of the racist patient. Am J Orthop (Belle Mead Nj) 2015;44(12):E477–9.

17. Paul-Emile K, Smith AK, Lo B, et al. Dealing with racist patients. N Engl J Med 2016;374(8):708–11.

18. Krebs EE, Garrett JM, Konrad TR. The difficult doctor? Characteristics of physicians who report frustration with patients: an analysis of survey data. BMC Health Serv Res 2006;6:128.

19. Lippa RA. Gender differences in personality and interests: when, where, and why? Soc Personal Psychol Compass 2010;4(11):1098–110.

20. Evaluation of humanistic qualities in the internist. Ann Intern Med 1983;99(5): 720–4.

21. Gabbard GO. The role of countertransference in contemporary psychiatric treatment. World Psychiatry 2020;19(2):243–4.

22. Heimann P. On counter-transference. Int J Psycho-anal 1950;31:81–4.

23. Halpern J. From idealized clinical empathy to empathic communication in medical care. Med Health Care Philos 2014;17(2):301–11.

24. Stienen MN, Scholtes F, Samuel R, et al. Different but similar: personality traits of surgeons and internists-results of a cross-sectional observational study. BMJ Open 2018;8(7):e021310.

25. Elder N, Ricer R, Tobias B. How respected family physicians manage difficult patient encounters. J Am Board Fam Med 2006;19(6):533–41.

26. Branch WT Jr. The road to professionalism: reflective practice and reflective learning. Patient Educ Couns 2010;80(3):327–32.

27. Sanyer ON, Fortenberry K. Using mindfulness techniques to improve difficult clinical encounters. Am Fam Physician 2013;87(6):402.

28. Airagnes G, Consoli SM, De Morlhon O, et al. Appropriate training based on Balint groups can improve the empathic abilities of medical students: a preliminary study. J Psychosom Res 2014;76(5):426–9.

29. Fiester A. The "difficult" patient reconceived: an expanded moral mandate for clinical ethics. Am J Bioeth 2012;12(5):2–7.

30. Strous RD, Ulman AM, Kotler M. The hateful patient revisited: relevance for 21st century medicine. Eur J Intern Med 2006;17(6):387–93.

31. Zurad EG. Don't be a target for a malpractice suit. Fam Pract Manag 2006;13(6): 57–64.

32. Schilling LM, Scatena L, Steiner JF, et al. The third person in the room: frequency, role, and influence of companions during primary care medical encounters. J Fam Pract 2002;51(8):685–90.

33. Onishi SL, Hebert RS. The Stanford prison experiment: implications for the care of the "difficult" patient. Am J Hosp Palliat Care 2016;33(1):64–8.

Using Technology to Enhance Communication

Matthew Sakumoto, MD, Raman Khanna, MD, MAS*

KEYWORDS

- Telemedicine • Telehealth communication • Health communication
- Doctor-patient relationship • Digital • Electronic health record

KEY POINTS

- A broad range of digital communication tools in health care exist, and choosing the right tool involves trade-offs between speed of message delivery and engagement with the message receiver.
- Patient-provider communication occurs through patient portals, open notes, and telehealth, and effective communication through these channels requires additional consideration due to a decrease in nonverbal cues.
- Digital provider-provider communication can help or hinder team-based care depending on the use of technology.
- Benefits of technology-enhanced communication include increased access/availability, asynchronous communication, improved data capture, and improved triage.
- Challenges to technology-assisted communication include widening the digital divide, concerns over security and privacy, and fragmentation of care and message burden.

Abbreviations	
EHR	Electronic Health Record
HITECH Act	Health Information Technology for Economic and Clinical Health Act
AVS	After Visit Summary
SMS	Short Message Service
PHI	Protected Health Information
HIPAA	Health Insurance Portability and Accountability Act

INTRODUCTION

Other than procedures, the vast majority of a provider's practice is communication. Whether speaking with a patient or a family member, writing notes in the chart, consulting a colleague, or ordering tests, medications, or referrals, communication is the

Department of Medicine, UCSF, San Francisco, CA, USA
* Corresponding author. 521 Parnassus Avenue, San Francisco, CA 94143-0131:
E-mail address: Raman.khanna@ucsf.edu

Med Clin N Am 106 (2022) 705–714
https://doi.org/10.1016/j.mcna.2022.01.010
0025-7125/22/© 2022 Elsevier Inc. All rights reserved.

through line for most clinical efforts.[1,2] The content, clarity, and correctness of these communications is extremely important; additionally, there are process considerations regarding how such communications are generated, transmitted, delivered, and consumed.

As clinical communication becomes predominantly, even overwhelmingly, digital, strategies for effective digital communication are a critical clinical skill. This article focuses on the processes for leveraging digital communication in the most efficient, secure, and clinically appropriate manner.

Background

Modes of health care communication

Digital communication tools exist in a range of media, with variable benefits and challenges in each. Broadly speaking, digital communication, much like its physical analogs, can occur synchronously (via audio or audiovisual connection) or asynchronously (via e-mail or secure chat). As shown in the communication hierarchy (**Fig. 1**), there is a trade-off between speed and engagement; some methods are very quick to produce and broadcast a message but less likely to engender a change in behavior or even a response from the recipient. Others take considerably more effort to create but better capture context and thus elicit engagement. To state things more bluntly, as in the analog world, messages that are cheap to send (such as bulk mail) are also cheap to ignore, whereas messages that are more expensive to send (such as hand-written, personalized cards) are also expensive to ignore. The reach of communication broadens from one-to-one at the top of this pyramid to one-to-many with more efficient modes of communication.

Targeted messaging via Web advertisements and e-mails is increasingly prevalent. Balancing this personalization is particularly important in optimizing the signal-to-noise ratio to make sure the message is received and interpreted in the intended manner.[3] This balance is important for patient-provider communication, as well as interprofessional communication between providers on the care team.

For example, automated health maintenance reminders (sent either physically or electronically) can reach a wide population, but may be filtered out by patients. The sender also matters, and patients are more likely to respond positively if the message comes from their provider over an anonymous bot.[4]

Patient-provider communication

Patient portal. The patient portal is a Web-based or mobile application that allows the patient to connect with portions of the electronic health record (EHR). Different portals vary in functionality but often include the ability to review medication lists and laboratory results, schedule appointments, and securely message with the care team.

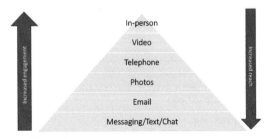

Fig. 1. Communication hierarchy.

Patient-provider messaging can also take the form of secure e-mail, voicemail/ phone call, and text messaging.[5] The content and "socioemotional tone" of text-based messaging is important to keep in mind, and voice inflection, facial cues, and nonverbal cues are lost in the text-only realm.[6]

Open notes. A decade-old experiment, the open-notes movement advocates for patients being able to read the clinical notes written about their care.[7] Research has shown that providers largely expected improved communication possibly at the expense of increased questions between visits, and patients ultimately found open notes to be very beneficial.[8] Remarkably, this benefit was greater for those with lower educational attainment.[9,10] Thanks to the 21st Century Cures Act, this promising experiment has overnight become the norm nationwide.[11] History and physical documents, discharge summaries, progress notes, and consultations have all gained a potent potential audience as patients gain the ability to observe the conversation about their care. However, it is not yet known whether the experiences of a few highly committed early institutions and their patients will generalize beyond their communities, or whether it will shrink rather than exacerbate the digital divide.[12]

Telehealth and Webside manner. Telehealth has increasingly become a mode of synchronous patient-provider communication; this includes both audio-only (phone call) and audiovisual (video visit) forms of telehealth. In the world of virtual care, there has been increasing recognition of Webside manner and digital body language.[13,14] There are specific skills and techniques for enhancing virtual communication: taking longer pauses to accommodate audio lag, placing the Web camera to maximize perceived eye contact and attention, and framing the field of view to include face and torso to capture nonverbal cues.[15] On the patient's side, it is also important to set expectations of focus and privacy. Telehealth offers increased health care access from the comfort of a patient's home, but unlike the clinic room, there are also limitations to privacy and distractions in the form of family members being nearby, or patients driving during their appointments. A summary of patient and provider suggestions is detailed in **Table 1**.

Provider-provider communication
The practice of medicine has become not only increasingly team based but also increasingly fragmented. In the past, the primary care provider would follow the patient's clinical course from the clinic, to the hospital, and back again, and radiology images were reviewed side-by-side in the reading room.[16] When paper charts were stored at the nurse's station, face-to-face communication occurred between the ordering provider and the nurse, or the provider would see the consultant as they placed their note into the chart binder. In the present, providers may be sequestered

Table 1
Telehealth and Webside manner

Recommendations for Providers	Recommendations for Patients
Take longer pauses to accommodate audio lag	Find a quiet, private space
Position web camera to maximize eye contact	Log on early to troubleshoot software or Internet connectivity
Frame face and torso to capture and convey nonverbal cues	Limit distractions such as family members, work, or driving during the virtual visit

into team rooms, coordinating care, charting, and sending orders, but separated from the rest of the care team.[17] Remote communication may increase the efficiency of communication, but may result in decreased interpersonal connection and missed nonverbal cues.

The note. Documentation in the medical record is the primary form of modern care team communication. The transition from paper charts to the EHR was primarily promoted by the HITECH Act of 2009 and EHR Incentive program (Meaningful Use, now called Promoting Interoperability program).[18] The main forms of documentation are the history and physical, daily progress note, consult note, and discharge summary; these serve as a one-to-many permanent record of the patient's clinical status, as well as the provider's thought process and recommendations for care. The discharge or transfer summary is a particularly important communication document, because it is often a summary of a complex hospital course, as the patient transitions to a different site of care, and different care team. Studies have shown that electronic discharge summaries significantly improve the quality and timeliness of the document,[19] and many organizations began autotransmitting these to the primary care provider as a way of satisfying the HITECH Act's Stage 1 of Meaningful Use.[20]

Team messaging. For "in the moment" communication, team members rely on phone calls, secure messaging via the EHR or a third-party application, Web paging, and e-mail.[21] In the inpatient setting a nurse may alert the care team to a deterioration in patient status. A pharmacist may message the ordering provider about a drug-drug interaction or dosage adjustment. Primary teams may message consultants to ask a clinical question and consultants may similarly reply with recommendations. In the ambulatory setting, these messages are for requests for refills, notification of a critical laboratory value, or even a notification that a patient is running late for their appointment. Some health systems have developed etiquette guides for secure messaging (**Fig. 2**). Nascent research on optimal communication strategies unsurprisingly suggests that including the reason for a communication and a preferred response method helps, but this remains to be better delineated.[22]

Current evidence

Availability and enrichment. The clinical note is very important for care team communication because it documents the current context and plan that arose at the time the note was finalized. The electronic clinical note has certain key benefits over paper: it is accessible anywhere, legible, and linked to other key information such as laboratory results and structured documentation from other clinicians.[23] Links and macros can pull in laboratory information and text from prior notes and can even autocalculate clinical risk scores for cardiac disease, strep throat, or pulmonary embolism augmenting the communication of the medical decision-making process. However, importing too much information can lead to note bloat, with some studies showing up to 50% of content copied from other sources.[24,25]

Asynchronous communication. The after visit summary (AVS) for patients provides a summary of the office visit or hospitalization, patient instructions and anticipatory guidance, and information on upcoming tests and future visits. The digital AVS can embed hyperlinks to Web-based resources to provide additional patient education, and even therapeutic options such as home-based physical therapy exercises. With the AVS available online via the patient portal, patients have timely and efficient access to their health information for managing health-related tasks.[26]

Secure Chat* — More urgent message. Need answer in minutes/hours. Text is not saved in chart. See Epic Secure Chat Rules of the Road for Priority Usage

	Secure Chat appropriate:	Secure Chat NOT appropriate
Provider->Staff	"Patient in exam room needs EKG" or vaccine, PAP or other ASAP coordination	"I was wondering ... " (too interruptive and low priority)
Staff->Provider	"Your next patient is here, how long might I tell them you will be?"	"Can you sign this in the next few days?"
Provider ->Provider	Contacting interpreting radiologist "Can you clarify this finding on your report? I have a Q..." Attach patient's chart "I have a patient here with me who needs to be seen today in your clinic"	"I saw your patient today and they are doing well, no concerns." (non-urgent)* "Thank you"
Operator ->Provider on call	"Mrs. Smith called and is having redness at her incision site, please call her back" Patient's chart will be attached	

***SECURE CHAT OK, IF REQUESTED OR PREFERRED BY CHAT RECIPIENT**

Staff Message — Less urgent. Need answer in days. Use as Reminder OR FYI OR Not related to specific patient. Text is not saved in chart but MAY BE discoverable.

	Staff Message appropriate	Staff Message NOT appropriate
Provider->Staff	"Please mail this letter I wrote, by tomorrow"	"I need you now in exam room ..." (too urgent, will NOT be seen quickly Use Secure Chat instead
Staff->Provider	Cindy's Birthday: cake in the break room today.	"This patient is so hateful." (discoverable, never appropriate)
Provider->Prov	Contacting radiologist "In general, can you order an MRI on pt with metal plate in c-spine?"	"Please review the CT scan on your patient and let me know how I should proceed." (needs to be in a phone or documentation only encounter NOT a staff message)
Provider-> Self	Reminder: to check on Pulm Nodule CT scan in 3 mo (remind me functionality " tickler")	"Please order a CBC, CMP, and a foot x-ray on my patient" (many things wrong with this, needs encounter with full order details)

Phone encounter** — Less urgent. Documents actions between visits in patient chart. **Doc only, telephone, quick note and orders only encounters all examples of these notes/encounters

	Phone Encounter/Note appropriate	Phone Encounter NOT appropriate
Provider->Staff	"Spoke with pt: no need to change med right now." "Please contact pt to come for urgent appt today."	"I don't like him, He is always late" (discoverable, never appropriate) "Husband wants a refill" (wrong patient chart)
Staff->Provider	"Pt with dysuria again; should she come for urine dip?"	"There's coffee and cake in the break room" Not appropriate in patient's chart
Provider->Prov For chart inclusion	"On call last night: Rx'd Z-pak on your patient." Called pt 3x in past 3 days, no answer, left message.	

Fig. 2. Examples of using Secure Chat versus other tools for clinical communication in clinic.

In addition to patient-provider communication, there has been an increase in secure messaging between health care professionals. The benefits of technology are the highly customized time lags allowed. Providers can respond right away to some questions, respond later if they need to look up information, or defer or redirect a message to another colleague; this allows everyone to perform at the top of their license. Furthermore, it is convenient to access these platforms from a smartphone. This team-based approach and EHR inbasket use facilitates providing better, more efficient, more timely patient care.[27] In the inpatient setting, messaging questions about symptoms and treatment plans are particularly important to patients and can improve length of stay and discharge planning.[28]

Improved data capture and triage. "Old" technology such as standardized question-naires, in combination with newer technology such as chatbots, can facilitate clinical triage and information collection without direct input from a health care provider. These tools can generate extra health care capacity and prevent unnecessary patient-generated messages, phone calls, and in-person visits by allowing patients to self-triage and self-schedule based on their symptoms.[29] Using the chat format (at a time when they are most focused on their health) can also have positive effects on their future health behaviors. This technology helps engage patients, provides them access to information, and helps them understand the implications of this information in a powerful moment of insight.[5]

Controversies

Technology can greatly enhance access and connectivity between the patients and the health care system. However, it is important to note some specific challenges that technology introduces.

Exacerbating inequality. Health and technological literacy can potentiate care in important ways, but as with many interventions, there is unfortunately a digital divide that must be minded. Many patients lack reliable access to smartphones, the Internet, or the use of services enabled through these mechanisms.[30] It is important to design any patient-facing technology with language, hearing or sight impairment, and Internet access in mind, or to provide alternative parallel options, such as phone call in addition to video visit.

Security and privacy. The introduction of digital communication workflows also intro-duces a key privacy trade-off, where patients can see far more of their information, but may also feel compelled or coerced into sharing it with their families. Patients cite pri-vacy and security concerns among the reasons that they do not use their online med-ical record.[31] Telehealth visits offer the convenience of receiving medical evaluation from home or the work office, but there are also new difficulties of finding a quiet, pri-vate space to conduct the visit.[32] Of note, several institutions struggled during the 21st Century Cures Act open notes implementation with how to practically prevent parents from reading adolescents' notes, especially when such notes sometimes contain sen-sitive information for which the adolescent might otherwise not seek care, and some ultimately settled on not allowing open notes at all during the patient's adolescent period.[33]

Fragmentation and message burden. Although the proliferation of patient portals, digital health applications, and digital resources on the patient side, and of various EHR and EHR-adjacent tools on the provider side, have tremendous potential to improve communication, they can also add to the complexity of care and commu-nication. Messages may be duplicated across multiple platforms, or they may be missed entirely. In addition, the lowered barriers to generating messages can lead to increased messaging burden, which is associated with provider burnout.[34]

Approach: practical guide to clinical communication in the tech-enabled world

To enhance benefits and mitigate challenges, the following are the practical con-siderations for a provider when thinking about technology and clinical communication:

1. *Each provider needs several nonoverlapping tools—no one tool (currently) covers all needs.* Most EHRs serve many needs described earlier, even if not perfectly: the creation of notes, the sharing of these notes with patients through portals,

slow asynchronous communication with specialists, and slow asynchronous communication with patients. Most providers and all inpatient settings, however, need an additional "fast" asynchronous platform for provider-to-provider communication, which can be met by a Short Message Service (SMS), but requires the cost of maintaining an independent directory and keeping all communication protected health information (PHI) free to avoid violating the Health Insurance Portability and Accountability Act (HIPAA), or by a dedicated tool. In addition, all providers need a mechanism for synchronous video and audio communication for video and audio visits. Phone visits are likely accommodated through a smartphone, perhaps with apps that mask the provider's phone number. Finally, all providers still need a fax number, mostly to be reachable by other providers who are still exclusively using fax machines, although this can be provided by the EHR in some cases and by an electronic vendor in other cases without the need for a true physical fax machine.

2. *When choosing vendors, providers negotiate trade-offs that go beyond price and features.* In general, EHR choice is not dictated by the availability of communication tools, so providers are left to manage whatever tools the chosen EHR makes available. On the other hand, providers may be heavily involved in the selection of the supplemental tools and will be considering price, the ability to maintain HIPAA compliance, video and audio quality, the ease of initiating or scheduling meetings, the ease of quickly onboarding a patient, the way of reaching patients who are not on smartphones or do not have access to audiovisual equipment, and so on. All are important considerations in their own right, and their importance varies depending on the patient population served and the services offered. An additional consideration may be what payors will reimburse. It is important for clinicians to learn how to identify and present communication technology solutions to their organization's internal advocates and champions.[35]

3. *Visits may be appropriate for in person, video, or audio only, and many may be appropriate for any modality.* A preexisting concern regarding the quality of video visits in the pre-COVID world has likely been laid to rest, or at least postponed, such that video visitation is no longer seen as "inferior" to in-person visitation but rather a fully appropriate alternative in many cases. The choice of in-person visitation versus video visitation should thus not be dictated by perceptions of inherent superiority but rather by practical considerations that make video visits or in-person visitation more appropriate in context. In-person visitation may be more appropriate for certain physical examination-sensitive conditions; however, video visits may actually be superior for patients who otherwise need to commute long distances, cannot take sufficient time off work, and/or need family members or others to be able to join the visit. Audio visits may be an acceptable alternative to either in many cases and have the benefit of being very quick to initiate. Patient preference plays an important and unpredictable role, and providers should be guided by patients when the aforementioned factors are not in play.

4. *Time makes up for touch.* When a provider cannot hold a patient's hand, the patient may find the connection less personal or more cold. Likewise, some physical and nonverbal cues may be less available. Providers can overcome these barriers by spending increased time developing rapport, eliciting a history, actively listening, and practicing "digital empathy" with the patient.[15] Video visits may even offer the opportunity for better eye contact, because providers can chart while talking into the Webcam, unlike some in-office configurations, where the provider's back is turned to the patient while typing.

5. *Select the correct tool for follow-up and between-visit consultation.* Patients attach a high emotional valence to the methods by which we reach them. Patients may be alarmed about a phone call, assuming it is bad news, but a phone call may also be interpreted as warmth and caring, particularly for an important follow-up. On the other hand, for most routine laboratory testing, digital communication is also routine and appropriate. Consider eliciting patient's preference for mode of follow-up communication.

6. *Communication is still the key part of tech-enabled communication.* This obvious point can be lost in the blizzard of platforms, technologies, and methodologies. Ultimately, communicating with our patients and with one another is not just a key obligation but a source of connection and professional satisfaction as well. All other considerations are secondary to making that connection and should not distract from it.

DISCUSSION

Clinical communication between providers and with patients is essential for safe, high-quality, and high-value care. Maximizing the technology-enabled benefits, while navigating potential pitfalls, requires picking the right communication tool for each situation. Providers also need to practice skills in digital empathy, including nonverbal and written communication with each other and with patients.

SUMMARY

Digital communication, facilitated by the rise of the EHR, by the launch of telehealth, and by the enormous acceleration wrought by the COVID-19 pandemic, has transformed clinical workflow. Much more than afterthoughts, each provider and provider group must think carefully about the tools they are using, the purposes to which they are being put, and the benefits, risks, and fault tolerance for each, before deciding on the correct choice in the moment and the correct choice globally for the needs of their practice. In this article, we have offered several suggestions on how to approach these important questions in tailoring one's practice and the practice of one's group. These new digital communication tools open the doors to novel care models to connect patients and providers. Most importantly, the message, not the medium, is the key to successful communication.

CLINICS CARE POINTS

- Familiarize yourself with multiple technology-enabled tools for communication because different patient groups and different clinical situations may require secure messaging versus a phone call or video visit.

- Set clear expectations and boundaries with patients for the different modes of inbound communication.

- To enhance virtual communication via video, consider your Webside manner: take longer pauses to accommodate audio lag, place the web camera to maximize perceived eye contact and attention, and have the patient step back to frame the field of view to include their face and torso to capture nonverbal cues.

- Consider improving between-visit messaging. When thoughtfully composed, asynchronous messaging between visits can help build rapport while also furthering the clinical care plan or screening for early symptoms.

DISCLOSURE

R. Khanna reports receiving licensing income from HillRom, Inc, which owns the Voalte product line. No HillRom or other products are mentioned in this article. M. Sakumoto reports past personal fees from PlushCare and Clearstep Health.

REFERENCES

1. Wachter RM. Annals for hospitalists inpatient notes - hospitalists and digital medicine-overcoming the productivity paradox. Ann Intern Med 2016;165(2): HO2-3.
2. Overhage JM, McCallie D. Physician time spent using the electronic health record during outpatient encounters. Ann Intern Med 2020;172(3):169–74.
3. Stanley D. Signal-to-noise, provider communication, and provider education. 2020. Available at: https://www.dirkstanley.com/2020/01/signal-to-noise-provider-communication.html. Accessed September 6, 2021.S.
4. Perri-Moore S, Kapsandoy S, Doyon K, et al. Automated Alerts and Reminders Targeting Patients: A Review of the Literature. Patient Educ Couns 2016;99(6): 953–9.
5. Kahn JS. A piece of my mind. Next: text. JAMA 2012;307(17):1807–8.
6. Hogan TP, Luger TM, Volkman JE, et al. Patient centeredness in electronic communication: evaluation of patient-to-health care team secure messaging. J Med Internet Res 2018;20(3):e82.
7. Delbanco T, Walker J, Bell SK, et al. Inviting Patients to read their doctors' notes: a quasi-experimental study and a look ahead. Ann Intern Med 2012;157(7):461–70.
8. Walker J, Leveille S, Bell S, et al. OpenNotes after 7 years: patient experiences with ongoing access to their clinicians' outpatient visit notes. J Med Internet Res 2019;21(5):e13876.
9. Gerard M, Chimowitz H, Fossa A, et al. The importance of visit notes on patient portals for engaging less educated or nonwhite patients: survey study. J Med Internet Res 2018;20(5):e191.
10. Bell SK, Roche SD, Mueller A, et al. Speaking up about care concerns in the ICU: patient and family experiences, attitudes and perceived barriers. BMJ Qual Saf 2018;27(11):928–36.
11. Federal rules mandating open notes. 2021. Available at: https://www.opennotes.org/onc-federal-rule/. Accessed October 8, 2021.
12. Ramsetty A, Adams C. Impact of the digital divide in the age of COVID-19. J Am Med Inform Assoc 2020;27(7):1147–8.
13. McConnochie KM. Webside manner: a key to high-quality primary care telemedicine for all. Telemed J E Health 2019;25(11):1007–11.
14. Schwartz D, DeMasi M. The importance of teaching virtual rapport-building skills in telehealth curricula. Acad Med 2021;96(9):1231–2.
15. Sakumoto M, Krug S. Enhancing digital empathy and reimagining the telehealth experience. Telehealth Medicine Today 2021;6(4). https://doi.org/10.30953/tmt.v6.304.
16. Wachter R. The digital doctor: hope, hype, and harm at the dawn of medicine's computer age. 1st edition. New York, NY: McGraw-Hill Education; 2017.
17. Verghese A. Culture shock — patient as icon, icon as patient. N Engl J Med 2008; 359(26):2748–51.
18. Adler-Milstein J, Jha AK. HITECH act drove large gains in hospital electronic health record adoption. Health Aff (Millwood) 2017;36(8):1416–22.

19. OLeary KJ, Liebovitz DM, Feinglass J, et al. Creating a better discharge summary: Improvement in quality and timeliness using an electronic discharge summary. J Hosp Med 2009;4(4):219–25. https://doi.org/10.1002/jhm.425.

20. CMS. medicare & medicaid EHR incentive program meaningful use stage 1 requirements overview. 2010. Available at: https://www.cms.gov/Regulations-and-Guidance/Legislation/EHRIncentivePrograms/downloads/mu_stage1_reqoverview.pdf. Accessed January 9, 2021.

21. Liu X, Sutton PR, McKenna R, et al. Evaluation of secure messaging applications for a health care system: a case study. Appl Clin Inform 2019;10(1):140–50.

22. Chu CD, Tuot DS, Harrison JD, et al. Completeness and quality of text paging for subspecialty consult requests. Postgrad Med J 2021;97(1150):511–4.

23. Airan-Javia S. Exemplars and Key Successes: CareAlign. Presented at: 25x5 Symposium; January 29, 2021; Virtual. https://www.dbmi.columbia.edu/25x5/. Accessed Feb 19, 2022.

24. Wang MD, Khanna R, Najafi N. Characterizing the source of text in electronic health record progress notes. JAMA Intern Med 2017;177:1212–3.

25. Hirschtick RE. Copy-and-Paste. JAMA 2006;295(20):2335–6.

26. Emani S, Healey M, Ting DY, et al. Awareness and use of the after-visit summary through a patient portal: evaluation of patient characteristics and an application of the theory of planned behavior. J Med Internet Res 2016;18(4):e77.

27. Jerzak J, Sinsky C. EHR In-Basket Restructuring for Improved Efficiency. Presented at: AMA Steps Forward; June 29, 2017. Available at: https://edhub.ama-assn.org/steps-forward/module/2702694. Accessed December 11, 2021.

28. Sieck CJ, Walker DM, Hefner JL, et al. Understanding secure messaging in the inpatient environment: a new avenue for communication and patient engagement. Appl Clin Inform 2018;9(4):860–8.

29. Judson TJ, Odisho AY, Neinstein AB, et al. Rapid design and implementation of an integrated patient self-triage and self-scheduling tool for COVID-19. J Am Med Inform Assoc 2020;27(6):860–6.

30. Lai J, Widmar NO. Revisiting the digital divide in the COVID-19 Era. Appl Econ Perspect Policy 2020. https://doi.org/10.1002/aepp.13104.

31. Patel V, Johnson, C. Individuals' use of online medical records and technology for health needs.; 2018:1-17.

32. Hall JL, McGraw D. For telehealth to succeed, privacy and security risks must be identified and addressed. Health Aff 2014;33(2):216–21.

33. UCSF MyChart - Login Page. 2021. Available at: https://ucsfmychart.ucsfmedicalcenter.org/ucsfmychart/Authentication/Login?mode=stdfile&option=faq#MF_diff. Accessed October 8, 2021.

34. Adler-Milstein J, Zhao W, Willard-Grace R, et al. Electronic health records and burnout: time spent on the electronic health record after hours and message volume associated with exhaustion but not with cynicism among primary care clinicians. J Am Med Inform Assoc 2020;27(4):531–8.

35. Sharp Index. Physician EHR Toolkit. Sharp Index. Available at: https://sharpindex.org/physician-ehr-toolkit. Accessed January 9, 2022.

Communicating with Community

Health Disparities and Health Equity Considerations

Sherrie Flynt Wallington, PhD, MA[a],*, Annecie Noel, DO[b]

KEYWORDS

- Theoretical frameworks • Health communication
- Community-based participatory research • Health literacy
- Communication technology • Health disparities • Community engagement
- Community communication strategies

KEY POINTS

- Community communication is crucial to addressing health disparities.
- Bidirectional and responsive communication builds trust and is more effective.
- Communication technology facilitates interactive communication.
- Access to communication technology is not equitably distributed.

INTRODUCTION

As communities grapple with the complexities of health disparities, particularly in the midst of the COVID-19 pandemic and the resulting deluge of health information and misinformation, effective communication is important at both the individual and community levels. This article explores many reasons why effective communication with communities is vital for the communities we serve.

Communication with communities can have a remarkable impact on community development and success.[1] Discussing community communication first calls for a definition of communication, as currently there is no single agreed on the definition of communication.[2] For the purposes of this discussion, we will use the definition, "Communication is the process of understanding and sharing meaning."[3] Using this definition in communications with communities can help clinicians and public health

[a] George Washington University, School of Nursing, 1919 Pennsylvania Avenue, Suite 500, Washington, DC 20048, USA; [b] Department of Medicine, Memorial Sloan Kettering Cancer Center, 1275 York Avenue, New York, NY 10065, USA
* Corresponding author.
E-mail address: sflyntwalling31@gwu.edu

Med Clin N Am 106 (2022) 715–726
https://doi.org/10.1016/j.mcna.2022.03.007
0025-7125/22/© 2022 Elsevier Inc. All rights reserved.

medical.theclinics.com

practitioners better understand the structural and socioeconomic pathways that promote and impede disparities.[4]

Community also needs a shared definition. The concept of community has been discussed and reformulated for many years.[5] We often use neighborhood units or sociodemographic measures to substitute for community.[6] While these definitions are useful for some populations,[7] many people identify with other communities, including their interests, workplace or occupation, cultural or ethnic communities, and communities of shared faith.[8,9] Attempts to methodically understand how people define community has given us this definition: "a group of people with diverse characteristics who are linked by social ties, share common perspectives, and engage in joint action in geographic locations or settings."[5] An important component of community is that of shared communication. How we communicate is deeply integrated in creating a shared experience and understanding.[7,8]

Before communicating with a community, it is important to understand the specifics of context, institutions, and boundaries.[5] There is an increasing awareness that communities need to be at the heart of efforts that seek to promote health.[9] What follows is not an exhaustive overview regarding communicating with communities. Rather, we share highlights of frameworks, strategies, and critical issues important to community communication.

APPROACH
Theoretic Frameworks for Communicating with Communities

There are many theoretic frameworks and models used in developing health communications for the purpose of understanding the relationships between information, on the one hand, and health-related behaviors and outcomes, on the other. These frameworks and models thereby support more effective communication development. While theories focus on influencing individual choice and intrapersonal processes,[10] following are a few that focus on communicating in a community context.

Social-ecological model
The social-ecological model (SEM)[11] illustrates relationships between layers of influence on individual health behavior decision making and actions. The model is a series of rings, with the Individual at the center, and each successive layer progressing outward into the world—Intrapersonal, Interpersonal, Organizational, Community, Policy.[12] SEM provides a structure for understanding multiple influential factors simultaneously, how those systems influence and interact with each other, and how structural systems impact cultural norms for groups.

Social determinants of health and structural influence model
In more recent years, a greater understanding of social determinants of health (SDOH) and their impact on health choices has been evolving.[13] The Structural Influence Model of Health Communication (SIM)[14] illustrates how SDOH interact with mediating and moderating conditions and impact health communication outcomes, leading to impact on health outcomes. SIM also calls attention to inequalities in communication and consequent inequalities in health. Important dimensions of communication inequality include: (a) access to and use of information channels and services, (b) attention to and processing of health information, and (c) capacity and ability to act on the information provided.

Community-based participatory research
There is growing interest in community-based participatory research (CBPR) to address health disparities.[15] Similar to patient-centered communication in a clinical

setting, CBPR involves an equal partnership between researchers and community partners, from study design and priority setting throughout the research process, to determining the dissemination of findings. This partnership yields a multi-faceted, in-depth, and practical solution while securing sustainable relationships with the community.[16] CBPR builds on traditional public health research methods, through the involvement of many different perspectives, resources, and skills, and facilitates learning for the researcher as well as the community members[17] to address historical obstacles to community partnerships (ie, skepticism, hostility).

Active community engagement continuum

The Active Community Engagement Continuum provides a model for assessing how engaged the community is. It measures engagement in 5 different areas of the communications development process: assessment, access to information, inclusion in decision making, efficacy of the local community's voice with institutions, and accountability of those institutions to the public. Each characteristic is measured on a scale: consultative, cooperative, collaborative.[18] The process is understood to be developed over time, as rapport and trust develop, and with each advance community members come closer to being change agents.

Just like patient-centered communication,[19] the most successful models for community communication facilitate rapport and trust building, increase understanding and knowledge all around, and incorporate logistical and contextual realities.[16] Interventions that lead to long-term relationships and increased understanding lead to longer lasting outcomes. Collectively, these aspects help elucidate critical issues facing communities such as technological advancements, trust, health literacy, and health disparities.

CONSIDERATIONS
Revolutions in Communication Technology

Communication technology provides the context and logistical options for communicating with communities, and each new technology promises better reach and more engagement. Medical and public health messaging traditionally consists of unilateral communications to persuade the public to adopt or adjust behaviors, in posters and print ads, in radio or video public service announcements.[20] These began in the 1800s with the earliest forms of mass communication for medical and public health, and have evolved with advances in mass media technologies.[20]

With the popularization of the Internet in the mid-1990s, medical and public health communications' possibilities expanded from one-size-fits-all directives.[21] Although the earliest webpages had the capacity to accept data and provide responses, early use of the new communication tools focused more often on static information strategies on the new platform. Expert-driven content for all audiences was similarly on websites as in print materials.[22] It has taken evolutions in theoretic frameworks for health communication to start using the full range of interactivity available from technology. Current medical and public health communications now have the potential to be interactive, tailored, and engaging on multiple levels. Tailoring communications (incorporating specific information that applies to the recipient) can draw from passively provided information or from information actively provided by the recipients.[23] Delivery formats include, for example, medical patient portals, interactive games,[24] question and answer,[25,26] synchronous and asynchronous interactions with a trained health guide,[25,26] or video conferencing for individual or group interactions.[25,26]

However, there are certain difficulties that have come with the new communication technologies. For example, across all aspects of information gathering, processing, and utilization, people report feeling overwhelmed, frustrated, and confused by the quantity of information available.[27] Exacerbating the impact of the quantity of information is the question of its quality. Misinformation (unintentionally misleading information) and disinformation (intentionally dishonest information) are becoming prominent issues in all aspects of information gathering and utilization.[28] Most people lack the skills to assess the reliability of well-designed mis/disinformation, and the quantity of information doesn't allow for deep assessment.[27,28]

Another challenge for health communicators is the fragmentation of mass media. In 1960, 90% of American households had a television, and most viewers had access to the "Big Three" national network channels plus a few local channels.[29] In 2000, only 32% of American households were still watching those 3 national networks, with much of the viewership shifting to the expanding cable networks,[30] and a cable customer could expect more than 100 channels in their basic package. In addition, in more recent years, Americans are getting their information from a wider variety of sources; online streaming of TV and previously cable channels, websites of news outlets and specific informational experts, and social media all compete with traditional television viewing.[31,32] This trend accelerated in 2020.[33] Current media consumption involves far more opting in on the part of the consumer, informational targeting of social media platforms, and diverging biases of many media producers.[34,35] Reaching significant audiences involves many more strategies than in previous generations.

Predictably, communication technology diffusion also suffers from disparities. Ownership of a desktop or laptop computer and having home broadband (high-speed Internet access) vary significantly by race and ethnicity.[36,37] Similar digital access divides exist between urban/suburban households, compared with rural,[38] and between Americans with a disability compared with those without.[39] Household income is another divider of Internet access; 92% of households that have $75,000 or more in annual income have broadband at home, compared with only 57% of households with lower than $30,000.[36] For many vulnerable households, Internet access is limited to a smartphone and cellular data or public Internet access.[40] These disparities in communication technologies also create disparities in information access,[41] which also contribute to health disparities.

Role of Trust in Communicating with Communities

The need for building trust with individual patients in clinical practice is well documented; without it, the benefits of health care access are profoundly limited.[42,43] The role of trust building in community communication is equally crucial to the impact of those measures. Lack of trust in public health research and organizations directly leads to a lack of participation in research, and access to health care, and thereby increased morbidity and mortality for underserved communities.[44–46] There are several benefits to building community partnerships in research and interventions, including having greater potential for sustained impact, community and individual cooperation, community empowerment to impact their health, and better informed funding and policies that are more likely to succeed.[47–49] In the case of risk communication in a crisis, it has been said that communication moves at the speed of trust. Without trust and clarity, the community cannot participate in the effort to contain the crisis, creating an opportunity for politicization, misinformation, and disinformation.[50] In the global emergency of COVID-19, we have seen how trust and lack of trust impact diagnostic testing, risk assessment and reduction, and treatment and vaccination

Timely, rapid response

Communications that come out quickly are perceived as more trustworthy than those that hesitate

Consistent and repetitive

Communications that repeat the information, explain it, and stay consistent are perceived as more trustworthy than those that change

Authentic, transparent

Communications that are honest about uncertainties and unknowns, that express empathy and shared experience are perceived as more trustworthy than those that are closed or unclear about the larger situation

Reciprocal and/or sustained relationships

Entities that have a history in the community, participating and giving back to the community are considered more trustworthy than those that show up and disappear

Not politicized

Communications and entities that are perceived as having political goals, as having politicized the topic of concern, or as having personal gain from the communications are perceived as less trustworthy

Fig. 1. Critical Components for Trust-Building Communications

efforts.[51] Across the trust-building research there are common themes, illustrated in **Fig. 1**.[52,53]

Health Literacy

Health literacy as a concept grew out of media literacy, which strives to understand and develop people's skills at accessing, assessing, and creating media and media messages.[54] Health literacy includes skills that enable people to access and understand health information, and apply the information to health-related decision-making.[55] In measuring health literacy, there are 3 basic areas to consider: functional health literacy (the ability to understand information), interactive health literacy (the ability to act on the information), and critical health literacy (the ability to assess and evaluate the information); see **Box 1**.[55]

Understanding the literacy level of a community and supporting increased health literacy are crucial aspects of successful communication.[56] In addition, health literacy has come to be understood as an SDOH and a mechanism by which socioeconomic status impacts health disparities.[57] Improved health literacy has been associated with the empowerment of communities and individuals in engaging with their health: increased and improved information seeking, care seeking, participation in shared decision-making, and health-related choices.[58] For individuals with chronic health conditions, health literacy skills seem to have a direct impact on one's capacity to manage their condition and navigate their treatment protocols.[59–62]

Box 1
Health literacy skills

Example: Diabetes Management
- Functional Health Literacy: Understand the terms and able to follow instructions
- Interactive Health Literacy: Make dietary choices based on guidelines, share in decision-making
- Critical Health Literacy: Evaluate new diabetes-related information for relevance and veracity

A significant number of health literacy interventions focus on providers and creators of health information increasing their skills in communicating with individuals with lower health literacy levels.[63] Fewer interventions are designed to increase the health literacy skills of the recipients of the information. When addressing health literacy skill development, most research measures improvement in condition-specific functional health literacy, with virtually no measurement of interactive or critical health literacy.[64] Teaching specific information, while easier to do within an intervention, provides fewer long-term benefits than developing skills. The few studies that have addressed interactive and critical health literacy involved complex study designs with multiple stages of learning.[65,66] These interventions adapt media literacy's skill development tools for health literacy, both in using interactive technologies and in addressing disparities in technology access and skills.[67]

Health Disparities

Health disparities are defined as systematic differences in health outcomes between groups of people or communities that are neither physiologically driven nor random.[68] Health disparities are often impacted by or intersect with SDOH.[69] SDOH include living with discrimination, living in poorly resourced areas and/or deeply polluted areas, detrimental work or housing conditions, among others.[69] These factors typically have a long history of impacting communities that persists into the present. An example of health disparities include increased infant mortality rates by race/ethnicity—Black infants are not weaker than White infants, but are impacted by their mothers and families living under racism; institutional and provider racism; and adverse social, economic, and environmental exposures.[70] In clinical practice, there has been a significant push to address health disparities through better patient–provider communication. The use of a comprehensive social history at intake is recommended to provide providers with SDOH information to better support patients.[71] Addressing cultural and contextual differences between providers and patients, for example, addressing provider biases, recognizing patient communication needs, and developing cultural safety or cultural competency training for providers, are other areas necessary to improve communications.[72–74]

Likewise, there has been significant effort in communication at the community level to address health disparities and SDOH. Areas of particular interest include adjusting communications for appropriate health literacy levels,[75] nuanced models of cultural appropriateness of messaging,[76] and addressing inequities in both access to online resources and in digital literacy.[77] Significant strategies and themes regarding quality health communication include: working with communities in developing plans and communications; comprehensive plans that address the complexity of the community context; culturally and linguistically appropriate communications; the roles of social support and social norms; community strengths as well as vulnerabilities; and institutional and environmental factors as facilitators or barriers to health behaviors.[78] It is important to note that clinical and community communications interact in addressing and exacerbating health disparities.[79]

Community Engagement

In addressing SDOH and health disparities, the expertise of the community is needed to develop effective communications and plans of action. One effective method of engaging the community is that of CBPR.[80] Community members are experts in how the health topic is discussed and understood, the factors that facilitate and prevent the desired outcome, and how the health topic fits into the community's larger context. In addition, the practice of engaging and working with the community provides the opportunity to build trust and understanding that can support a sustainable impact.[81] CBPR has been shown to be effective in a wide variety of health concerns,[82–85] and across a variety of communities.[82,84–87]

However, CBPR and community engagement still have challenges to overcome to be most effective. The two most cited reasons for communities to distrust researchers are: (a) power imbalance in the process;[88] and (b) lack of tangible benefits for the community.[89] In practice, it is common for researchers to engage community members after the fundamental decisions are made surrounding priorities and methods. Practitioners and researchers then approach communities, holding on to the resources and power in the relationship. This both diminishes trust and limits the contributions of the community expertise.[90] Afterward, it is common for dissemination to be mostly or completely limited to academic publication, with limited benefit for the community that participated.[89] Addressing these limitations involves authentic engagement with the community from the outset, defining and practicing values, and embracing accountability when falling short of those goals.[90] Developing community communication in a CBPR framework requires a commitment to the community, and holds the best promise for making those communications impactful.

SUMMARY

As the models for addressing health disparities demonstrate, individuals exist in the context of their physical and social communities, making communicating with communities crucial to ameliorating health disparities. Communication works best when it is bidirectional and responsive. Recent advancements in communications technology make responsive community communication easier to achieve than previously possible, although they come with caveats and disadvantages—access is not as universal or equitably distributed as is needed, and misinformation and trust issues are more complicated in the age of digital literacy. At the same time, engaging the community with authentic, reciprocal, sustained relationships is the most effective way to both reach and understand the community.

CLINICS CARE POINTS

Based on research in CBPR and health communication, we suggest these strategies for communicating with communities.[91–93]

- *Listen to the community*: Effective communications must be specific to the needs, language, context, and priorities of the community. The first step is to listen to the community.
- *Build equitable partnerships*: Trust is earned with sustained, reciprocal relationships, and partnerships that are not equitable lose trust. Valuing and honoring partnerships is crucial to success.
- *Contribute to the community*: The intervention should give back to the community in a way that is meaningful to the recipients. This could be capacity building, information sharing, or material/logistical benefits.
- *Speak the same language*: Use the same language the community does in communications. Demonstrate having heard and respected what the community shared.

DISCLOSURE

The authors have nothing to disclose.

REFERENCES

1. Aruma EO. Roles of communication in community development. Int J Netw Commun Res 2018;5(1):1–10.

2. Dance, Frank E.X. "What Is Communication?: Nailing Jello to the Wall." Association for Communication Administration Bulletin 48.4 (1984): 4–7. Print.

3. Pearson J, Nelson P. An introduction to human communication: understanding and sharing. Boston (MA): McGraw-Hill; 2000. p. 6.

4. National Academies of Sciences, Engineering, and medicine. Communities in action: pathways to health equity. Washington (DC): The National Academies Press; 2017. https://doi.org/10.17226/24624.

5. MacQueen KM, McLellan E, Metzger DS, et al. What is community? An evidence-based definition for participatory public health. Am J Public Health 2001;91(12): 1929–38.

6. Green LW, Ottoson JM. 8th edition. Community and population health, 4. Boston (MA): WCB/McGraw-Hill; 1999. p. 41–2.

7. Chavis DM, Lee K. What is community anyway?. Available at: https://ssir.org/articles/entry/what_is_community_anyway#. Accessed February 15, 2022.

8. Thomas J, McDonagh D. Shared language: toward more effective communication. Australas Med 2013;6(1):46–54.

9. Sanders Thompson VL, Ackermann N, Bauer KL, et al. Strategies of community engagement in research: definitions and classifications. Transl Behav Med 2021;11(2):441–51.

10. Cameron KA. A practitioner's guide to persuasion: an overview of 15 selected persuasion theories, models and frameworks. Patient Educ Couns 2009;74(3): 309–17.

11. Prochaska JO, DiClemente CC. Stages of change in the modification of problem behaviors. In: Hersen M, Eisler RM, Miller PM, editors. Progressing behaviors modification. Sycamore (IL): Sycamore Press; 1992. p. 184–214.

12. Glanz K, Melvin C. How not to get lost in translation: implementing the recommendations and identifying research gaps. Am J Prev Med 2008;35(1 Suppl):S3–5.

13. US Department of Health and Human Services, Office of disease prevention and health promotion. Healthy People 2030: Social Determinants of Health. Available at: https://health.gov/healthypeople/objectives-and-data/social-determinants-health. Accessed February 6, 2022.

14. Viswanath K, Kreuter MW. Health disparities, communication inequalities, and eHealth: a commentary. Am J Prev Med 2007;32(5):S131–5.

15. D'Alonzo KT. Getting started in CBPR: Lessons in building community partnerships for new researchers. Nurs Inq 2010;17(4):282–8.

16. Israel BA, Coombe CM, Cheezum RR, et al. Community-based participatory research: A capacity-building approach for policy advocacy aimed at eliminating health disparities. Am J Public Health 2010;100(11):2094–102.

17. Schulz AJ, Israel BA, Coombe CM, et al. A community-based participatory planning process and multilevel intervention design: toward eliminating cardiovascular health inequities. Health Promot Pract 2011;12(6):900–11.

18. Agency for Toxic Substances and Disease Registry. Chapter 1: Models and Frameworks for the Practice of Community Engagement. In: ATSDR. Principles of community engagement. Washington (DC): NIH Publication No; 2015. p. 11–7782.

19. King A, Hoppe RB. Best Practice" for Patient-Centered Communication: a narrative review. J Graduate Med Educ 2013;385–93.

20. Salmon CT, Poorisat T. The rise and development of public health communication. Health Commun 2020;35(13):1666–77.

21. Rogers S. The role of technology in the evolution of communication. Forbes 2019. Available at: https://www.forbes.com/sites/solrogers/2019/10/15/the-role-of-technology-in-the-evolution-of-communication/. Accessed February 5, 2022.

22. Khanzode CA, Sarode RD. Evolution of the world wide web: From Web 1.0 to 6.0. Intern J Digital Libr Serv 2016;2:1–11.

23. Kreuter M, Farrell D, Olevitch L, et al. Tailoring health messages: customizing communication with computer technology. Mahawh (NJ): Lawrence Erlbaum Associates; 2000.

24. Sharifzadeh N, Kharrazi H, Nazari E, et al. Health education serious games targeting health care providers, patients, and publich health users: scoping review. JMIR Serious Games 2020;8(1):e13459.

25. Healthy People 2020: Health communication and health information technology. Available at: https://www.healthypeople.gov/2020/topics-objectives/topic/health-communication-and-health-information-technology. Accessed February 6, 2022.

26. Patmon FL, Gee PM, Rylee TL, et al. Using interactive patient engagement technology in clinical practice: a qualitative assessment of nurses' perceptions. J Med Internet Res 2016;18(11):e298.

27. Viswanath K, Nagler RH, Bigman-Galimore CA, et al. The communications revolution and health inequalities in the 21st century: implications for cancer control. Cancer Epidemiol Biomarkers Prev 2012;21(10):1701–8.

28. Hwang Y, Ryu JY, Jeong SH. Effects of disinformation using Deepfake: The protective effect of media literacy education. Cyberpsychology, Behav Social Networking 2021;24(3):188–93.

29. Blanks Hindman D, Wiegand K. The big three's prime-time decline: a technology and social context. J Broadcasting Electron Media 2008;52(1):119–35.

30. The Rise of Cable Television. Television in American Society Reference Library. Available at: https://www.encyclopedia.com/arts/news-wires-white-papers-and-books/rise-cable-television. Accessed February 6, 2022.

31. The State of Traditional TV with Q3 2020 Data. Marketing Charts. 2021. Available at: https://www.marketingcharts.com/featured-105414. Accessed February 5, 2022.

32. More than eight-in-ten Americans get their news from digital devices. Pew Research Center. 2021. Available at: https://www.pewresearch.org/fact-tank/2021/01/12/more-than-eight-in-ten-americans-get-news-from-digital-devices/. Accessed February 5, 2022.

33. Green R. New report finds 1.3 million new users joined social media every day during 2020. Campaign Brief. 2021. Available at: https://campaignbrief.com/new-report-finds-1-3-million-new-users-joined-social-media-every-day-during-2020/. Accessed February 5, 2022.

34. Cinelli M, de Francisci Morales G, Galeazzi A, et al. The echo chamber effect on social media. PNAS 2021;118(9). e2023301118.

35. Lewis-Hughes J. Disinformation and social media: a threat to security and peace. 2019. Available at: https://theowp.org/reports/disinformation-and-social-media-a-threat-to-security-and-peace/. Accessed February 6, 2022.

36. Internet/Broadband Fact Sheet. Pew Research Center. 2021. Available at: https://www.pewresearch.org/internet/fact-sheet/internet-broadband/. Accessed February 5, 2022.

37. Atske S, Perrin A. Home broadband adoption, computer ownership vary by race, ethnicity in the U.S. Pew Research Center. 2021. Available at: https://www.pewresearch.org/fact-tank/2021/07/16/home-broadband-adoption-computer-ownership-vary-by-race-ethnicity-in-the-u-s/. Accessed February 5, 2022.

38. Vogels EA. Some digital divides persist between rural, urban, and suburban America. Pew Research Center. 2021. Available at: https://www.pewresearch.org/fact-tank/2021/08/19/some-digital-divides-persist-between-rural-urban-and-suburban-america/. Accessed February 5, 2022.

39. Perrin A, Atske S. Americans with disabilities less likely than those without to own some digital devices. Pew Research Center. 2021. Available at: https://www.pewresearch.org/fact-tank/2021/09/10/americans-with-disabilities-less-likely-than-those-without-to-own-some-digital-devices/. Accessed February 5, 2022.

40. Anderson M, Horrigan JB. Smartphones help those without broadband get online, but don't necessarily bridge the digital divide. Pew Research Center. 2016. Available at: https://www.pewresearch.org/fact-tank/2016/10/03/smartphones-help-those-without-broadband-get-online-but-dont-necessarily-bridge-the-digital-divide/. Accessed February 5, 2022.

41. Ramanadhan S, Viswanath K. Health and the information nonseeker: A profile. Health Commun 2006;2:131–9.

42. Asan O, Yu Z, Crotty BH. How clinician-patient communication affects trust in health information sources: temporal trends from a national cross-sectional survey. PLoS One 2021;16(2):e0247583.

43. Street RL Jr, Makoul G, Arora NK, et al. How does communication heal? Pathways linking clinician-patient communication to health outcomes. Patient Educ Couns 2009;74(3):295–301.

44. Hudson KL, Lauer MS, Collins FS. Toward a new era of trust and transparency in clinical trials. JAMA 2016;316(13):1353–4.

45. Holroyd TA, Oloko OK, Salmon DA, et al. Communicating recommendations in public health emergencies: the role of public health authorities. Health Secur 2020;18(1):21–8.

46. Romanelli M, Hudson KD. Individual and systemic barriers to health care: Perspectives of lesbian, gay, bisexual, and transgender adults. Am J Orthopsychiatry 2017;87(6):714–28.

47. Wolff M, Bates T, Beck B, et al. Cancer prevention in underserved African American communities: barriers and effective strategies – a review of the literature. WMJ 2003;102(5):36–40.

48. Ahmed SA, Beck B, Maurana CA, et al. Overcoming barriers to effective community-based participatory research in US medical schools. Educ Health (Abingdon) 2004;17(2):141–51.

49. Dobransky-Fasiska D, Brown C, Pincus HA, et al. Developing a community-academic partnership to improve recognition and treatment of depression in underserved African American and white elders. Am J Geriatr Psychiatry 2009; 17(11):953–64.

50. van Zoonen W, van der Meer T. The importance of source and credibility perception in times of crisis: crisis communication in a socially mediated era. J Public Rel Res 2015;27(5):371–88.

51. Willis DE, Andersen JA, Bryant-Moore K, et al. COVID-19 vaccine hesitancy: Race/ethnicity, trust, and fear. Clin Transl Sci 2021;14(6):2200–7.

52. Dancy BL, Wilbur J, Talashek M, et al. Community-based research: Barriers to recruitment of African Americans. Nurs Oulook 2004;52(5):234–40.

53. Timmerman GM. Addressing barriers to health promotion in underserved women. Fam Community Health 2007;30(1 Suppl):S34–42.

54. Baker FW. History of media literacy. In: Silverblatt A, editor. The praeger handbook of media literacy. Santa Barbara (CA): ABC CLIO; 2013. Available at:

https://www.frankwbaker.com/mlc/media-literacy-history/. Accessed February 10, 2022.

55. Liu C, Wang D, Liu C, et al. What is the meaning of health literacy? A systematic review and qualitative synthesis. Fam Med Commun Health 2020;8:e000351.

56. Kreps GL, Neuhauser L, Sparks L, et al. Promoting convergence between health literacy and health communication. Stud Health Technol Inform 2020;269:526–43.

57. Nutbeam D, Lloyd JE. Understanding and responding to health literacy as a social determinant of health. Annu Rev Public Health 2021;42:159–73.

58. Jorm AF. Mental health literacy: empowering the community to take action. for better mental health. Am Psychol 2012;67(3):231–43.

59. Kim MT, Kim KB, Ko J, et al. Health literacy and outcomes of a community-based self-help intervention: A case of Korean Americans with type 2 diabetes. Nurs Res 2020;69(3):210–8.

60. Kim H, Goldsmith JV, Sengupta S, et al. Mobile health application and e-health literacy: Opportunities and concerns for cancer patients and caregivers. J Cancer Educ 2019;34(1):3–8.

61. Marciano L, Camerini AL, Schulz PJ. The role of health literacy in diabetes knowledge, self-care, and glycemic control: a meta-analysis. J Gen Intern Med 2019; 34(6):1007–17.

62. Cajita MI, Cajita TR, Han HR. Health literacy and heart failure: a systematic review. J Cardiovasc Nurs 2016;31(2):121–30.

63. Coleman C. Health literacy and clear communication best practices for telemedicine. Health Lit Res Pract 2020;4(4):e224–9.

64. Nutbeam D, McGill B, Premkumar P. Improving health literacy in community populations: A review of progress. Health Promot Int 2018;33(5):901–11.

65. Conard S. Best practices in digital health literacy. Int J Cardiol 2019;292:277–9.

66. McCormack L, Thomas V, Lewis MA, et al. Improving low health literacy and patient engagement: A social ecological approach. Patient Educ Couns 2017; 100(1):8–13.

67. Levin-Zamir D, Bertschi I. Media health literacy, eHealth literacy, and the role of the social environment in context. Int J Environ Res Public Health 2018;15:1643.

68. Krieger N. A glossary for social epidemiology. J Epidemiol Community Health 2001;55(10):693–700.

69. World Health Organization. Social Determinants of Health. Available at: https://www.who.int/health-topics/social-determinants-of-health. Accessed February 18, 2022.

70. Willis E, McManus P, Magallanes N, et al. Conquering racial disparities in perinatal outcomes. Clin Perinatol 2014;41(4):847–75.

71. Adler NE, Stead WW. Patients in context—EHR capture of social and behavioral determinants of health. Obstet Gynecol Surv 2015;70(6):388–90.

72. Pérez-Stable EJ, El-Toukhy S. Communicating with diverse patients: how patient and clinician factors affect disparities. Patient Educ Couns 2018;101(12): 2186–94.

73. Kiles TM, Cernasev A, Leibold C, et al. Patient perspectives of discussing social determinants of health with community pharmacists [published online ahead of print, 2022 Jan 17]. J Am Pharm Assoc (2003) 2022. S1544-3191(22)00007-3.

74. Curtis E, Jones R, Tipene-Leach D, et al. Why cultural safety rather than cultural competency is required to achieve health equity: a literature review and recommended definition. Int J Equity Health 2019;18(1):174.

75. Schillinger D. The intersections between social determinants of health, health literacy, and health disparities. Stud Health Technol Inform 2020;269:22–41.

76. Tan NQP, Cho H. Cultural appropriateness in health communication: a review and a revised framework. J Health Commun 2019;24(5):492–502.

77. Viswanath K, Kreuter MW. Health disparities, communication inequalities, and e-Health: A commentary. Am J Prev Med 2007;32(5 Suppl):S131–3.

78. Schiavo R. Health Communication in Health Disparities Settings. J Community Health 2014;7(2):71–3.

79. Horowitz C, Lawlor EF. Appendix D: Community Approaches to Addressing Health Disparities. In Institute of Medicine (US) Roundtable on Health Disparities (eds). Challenges and Successes in Reducing Health Disparities: Workshop Summary. Available at: https://www.ncbi.nlm.nih.gov/books/NBK215366/. Accessed February 18, 2022.

80. Leung MW, Yen IH, Minkler M. Community based participatory research: a promising approach for increasing epidemiology's relevance in the 21st century. Int J Epidemiol 2004;33(3):499–506.

81. Springer MV, Skolarus LE. Community-based participatory research: Partnering with communities. PMC 2019;50(3):e48–50.

82. Joseph JJ, Nolan TS, Williams A, et al. Improving cardiovascular health in black men through a 24-week community-based team lifestyle change intervention: The black impact pilot study. Am J Prev Cardiol 2022;9:100315.

83. Rodriguez Espinosa P, Verney SP. The underutilization of community-based participatory research in psychology: a systematic review. Am J Community Psychol 2021;67(3–4):312–26.

84. Nash SH, Greenley R, Dietz-Chavez D, et al. Incorporating participant and clinical feedback into a community-based participatory research study of colorectal cancer among alaska native people. J Community Health 2020;45(4):803–11.

85. Ma GX, Toubbeh JI, Su X, et al. ATECAR: An Asian American community-based participatory research model on tobacco and cancer control. Health Promot Pract 2004;5(4):382–94.

86. Nicolaidis C, Raymaker D, Katz M, et al. Community-based participatory research to adapt health measures for use by people with developmental disabilities. Prog Community Health Partnersh 2015;9(2):157–70.

87. Strang JF, Knauss M, van der Miesen A, et al. A clinical program for transgender and gender-diverse neurodiverse/autistic adolescents developed through community-based participatory design. J Clin Child Adolesc Psychol 2021;50(6):730–45.

88. Roura M. The social ecology of power in participatory health research. Qual Health Res 2021;31(4):778–88.

89. Chen PG, Diaz N, Lucas G, et al. Dissemination of results in community-based participatory research. Am J Prev Med 2010;39(4):372–8.

90. Alang S, Batts H, Letcher A. Interrogating academic hegemony in community-based participatory research to address health inequities. J Health Serv Res Policy 2021;26(3):215–20.

91. Ward M, Schulz AJ, Israel BA, et al. A conceptual framework for evaluating health equity promotion within community-based participatory research partnerships. Eval Program Plann 2018;70:25–34.

92. Hicks S, Duran B, Wallerstein N, et al. Evaluating community-based participatory research to improve community-partnered science and community health. Prog Community Health Partnersh 2012;6(3):289–99.

93. Mackert M, Table B, Yang J, et al. Applying Best Practices from Health Communication to Support a University's Response to COVID-19. Health Commun 2020;35(14):1750–3.

Improving Communication Skills

A Roadmap for Humanistic Health Care

Andrew A. Chang, MD, MPH, MA[a],*, Caitlin H. Siropaides, DO[b],
Calvin L. Chou, MD, PhD[c]

KEYWORDS

- Communication • Learning • Teaching • Feedback • Motivation • Bias • Leadership

KEY POINTS

- Communication skills can be learned, practiced, and mastered. Key foundational micro-skills of communication have broad applicability and utility across various roles in health care.
- Understanding the factors and types of motivation in behavior change can affect the approach toward communication skill improvement.
- Central to ongoing improvement in communication skills is personal awareness, which includes recognition of bias and emotional reactions, their behavioral consequences, and how to intervene when necessary.
- Methods to improve communication skills depend on psychological safety, coaching with directed feedback (individually or in groups), institutional support, and a culture of continuous learning.

INTRODUCTION

Providers must communicate clearly and effectively when working with patients and teams in our complex health care system. Many communication skills can be developed and honed, including creating rapport, setting an agenda, eliciting the patient's perspective, naming and managing emotion, providing information, checking for understanding, and collaborating on treatment plans. Studies show that effective use of communication skills leads to improved patient outcomes, patient and clinician satisfaction, and institutional metrics.[1,2] However, it may be difficult to know where

[a] Department of Medicine, State University of New York Downstate, NYC Health + Hospitals/ Kings County, 451 Clarkson Avenue, E Building 7th Floor Adult Primary Care, Brooklyn, NY 11203, USA; [b] Department of Internal Medicine, Section of Supportive and Palliative Care, University of Texas Southwestern Medical Center, 5323 Harry Hines Boulevard, Dallas, TX 75390, USA; [c] Department of Medicine, University of California and Veterans Affairs Healthcare System, VA Medical Center, 4150 Clement St (136MP), San Francisco, CA 94121, USA
* Corresponding author.
E-mail address: changa3@nychhc.org

Med Clin N Am 106 (2022) 727–737
https://doi.org/10.1016/j.mcna.2022.01.011
0025-7125/22/© 2022 Elsevier Inc. All rights reserved.

to start, because effective communication is a complex series of interactions that involve preparation, receptivity, self-awareness, management of emotions in oneself and in others, as well as content expertise.

For optimal learning of any new skill, thoughtful learners might identify smaller, more achievable "parts" to make up the whole. Similarly, clinicians can approach communication as a set of skills, or "microskills", some of which are listed in **Box 1**. In addition, cognitive frameworks (see **Box 1**) provide explicit processes for common communication exchanges and help to identify the common landmarks of a conversation. Although this approach might seem robotic and contradictory to authentic communication, cognitive frameworks take the guesswork out of interactions. Instead, they allow for more freedom to connect with a patient using authentic responses and styles while relying on evidence-based skill sets that can offload those internal worries. Understanding and envisioning the larger flow of a conversation enables people to identify where they are in the conversation and intentionally practice new expressions to enrich their authentic style.

Here we outline a sampling of these frameworks that enable health care providers to take steps to improve their health care communication skills. We begin with discussing the intrinsic and extrinsic motivators to improving communication skills. We continue with a review of foundational communication microskills and suggestions on how to improve them through the perspectives of the clinician as a self-learner, the clinician with external coaching, and the administrator/leader. We hope that highlighting the evidence and applicability of these foundational skills provides relevance and context on this journey toward improved communication skills.

BACKGROUND: SUPPORTING MOTIVATION TO IMPROVE COMMUNICATION SKILLS

Motivation to improve underlies any behavior change. When a clinician commits to change, either via intrinsic or extrinsic motivation, they can access the underlying building blocks for effective learning. In health care communication, these fundamentals include awareness of self ("personal awareness") and skill in eliciting another's emotions and perspective (perspective-taking). As people exchange information, dialogue progresses as a dynamic interplay of emotions and reactions for all involved. Developing expertise in communication skills, as with any skill, requires deliberate practice, reflection, and coaching through feedback with motivation as the ultimate starting point.[3,4]

Box 1	
Explanation of microskills and cognitive frameworks	
Term	**Definition**
Microskills of communication	Specific competencies for communicating effectively with others. In addition to these largely externally displayed and objectively measurable skills, additional skills reflect one's internal thoughts about and processing of communication as it occurs in the moment: these include personal awareness, recognition and mitigation of biases, and appreciation of emotion
Cognitive frameworks	A collection of microskills that share a common purpose or goal, which provide explicit processes for common communication exchanges, and common landmarks of a conversation. (ie, internal conversation/ commentary about how much time is left in a visit, jumping to conclusions, making biased assumptions)

Motivation to improve is a spectrum, with the intrinsically self-motivated at one end ("I want to do this") and the extrinsically motivated at the other ("I'm being forced to do this"). Strategies to augment motivation vary across this spectrum. Although readers of this article may already have higher levels of intrinsic motivation around communication skill development, it is instructive to examine the theoretic underpinnings of motivation.

Self-Determination Theory postulates that satisfying innate psychological needs for *relatedness*, *competence*, and *autonomy* enhances self-motivation and mental health (**Table 1**).[5,6] Clarifying these underlying needs as they relate to communication skills may inspire learners toward further growth.

Intrinsic Motivation

For the self-motivated clinician, tools abound (eg, self-reflection, deliberate practice, communication skills courses, independent reading). Taking personal inventory of challenges in communication guides practice and intention building for continuous quality improvement. The more intrinsically motivated the provider, the more they will enjoy the challenges of learning increasingly complex skills. Subsequent sections will delve deeper into these tools.

Extrinsic Motivation

The goal of extrinsic motivation is to build toward and enhance intrinsic motivation for long-lasting impact (see **Table 1**). Verbal positive reinforcement, similar to praise, has an enhancing effect on motivation, particularly if the praise is unexpected[8] or if focused on behavior rather than characteristics, which may perpetuate a fixed mind-set.[9] On the other hand, numerous studies have shown that tangible extrinsic rewards

Table 1
Factors and types of motivation for clinicians, adapted from Self-Determination Theory[5,6]

		Definition	Example of how communication skills can relate to factors or types of motivation
Motivation Factors	*Relatedness*	A need to develop meaningful interactions with others.	A disconnecting conflict with a patient that continues to gnaw at a provider can impel them to enhance their communication skills.
	Competence	The perceived ability to master and achieve.	Effective communication skills can improve interpersonal interactions and outcomes.[7]
	Autonomy	The opportunity to control one's actions.	Using agenda-setting skills can improve predictability in encounters.
Motivation Types[6]	*Intrinsic*	The inherent tendency to seek out novelty and challenges, to extend and exercise one's capacities, to explore, and to learn.	Interest and challenges are inherent in the activity of communication skill development.
	Extrinsic	The performance of an activity in order to attain some external outcome.	A health care provider is mandated to take a communication training due to low patient satisfaction ratings.

such as money or gifts can damage intrinsic motivation.[10] When an expectation of a tangible extrinsic reward has been set and then removed or not applied equally, motivation decreases.[11] Although there is some controversy around these studies, extrinsic motivation can influence intrinsic motivation.[12] For example, monetary incentives supporting COVID-19 vaccination may induce those who have low motivation to receive the vaccine; however, anyone already vaccinated without the monetary incentive may feel slighted or excluded. A subset may be even less likely to obtain vaccination without additional tangible rewards.

BACKGROUND: FOUNDATIONAL MICROSKILLS FOR EFFECTIVE COMMUNICATION

Foundational microskills for effective communication in health care comprise a cognitive framework that has wide applicability. The major domains of the microskills include (1) handling one's own emotions through personal awareness and bias recognition, (2) perspective-taking and understanding the other's emotions, and (3) sharing information (**Table 2**).

Deepening Personal Awareness

Personal awareness is the recognition of how one's emotional reactions influence behaviors. Deepening personal awareness involves becoming mindful of one's own emotional reactions, then recognizing whether the behaviors that follow meet the needs of the patient. The stimuli and their emotional responses vary widely for everyone. Common unrecognized feelings include fear of losing control, addressing psychological issues, or appearing unpleasant. Common unrecognized resultant behaviors include overcontrolling the interview (eg, interrupting, changing the subject), avoidance, or superficial handling of the issue.[13] As an example, a patient is suffering from depression and asking for help. If the clinician was raised in a culture valuing stoicism, the clinician may feel uncomfortable (personal emotional reaction). Behaviorally, the clinician may change the subject to avoid engaging with the issue (inappropriate behavioral consequence), leaving the patient without the needed assistance. After recognizing emotional reactions, the next step is to change maladaptive behavioral responses to helpful ones that match the patient's needs. This process requires honesty with oneself and may be best facilitated with a trained coach.

Improving Recognition of Bias

Bias is related to personal awareness and especially salient, as health care providers work to reduce disparities and improve diversity, equity, and inclusion. In communication, attachment to one's personal agenda or biases risks blocking connection to the patient and understanding of their perspective. Using self-awareness, clinicians can

Table 2
Foundational microskills for effective communication

Major Domain		Examples of communication microskills
Handling one's own emotions	Personal awareness[13]	Recognition of emotional reactions Recognition of behavioral consequences
	Bias recognition	Self-reflection Implicit Association Test (IAT)[14]
Perspective-taking		Agenda setting[15] Open-ended questions[16]
Sharing information[17]		Ask-Respond-Tell (ART) Model Teach-back

recognize the presence of bias and withhold judgment, both of which are necessary steps before using perspective-taking (see later discussion) to tailor their recommendations to better meet patient needs; this has the added benefit of reducing conflict and increasing both patient and clinician satisfaction.

Not all biases are in one's awareness. Unconscious or implicit bias is another type of blind spot that limits the ability to grow one's communication skills. These more insidious forms of bias are unfortunately common, particularly around race. Researchers at Harvard University have developed Implicit Association Tests to uncover—but not cure—unconscious bias.[18] Once revealed, the provider must incorporate that information into their awareness to improve further. Deliberate practice is needed to work through mitigating bias.

Enhancing Perspective-Taking

Similar to self-awareness of personal emotions, recognition of others' emotions is crucial to effective communication. Perspective-taking is a foundational microskill that elicits patient emotion and informs how best to share information and action plan collaboratively. It is the basis of advanced skill frameworks, including relationship-centered interviewing, motivational interviewing, nonviolent communication, and professionalism remediation.[19–22] When done effectively, perspective-taking removes assumptions about others' feelings, thoughts, and actions and allows for deepened understanding of an individual's nuanced personal needs and values. This strategy is called individuation, a process that evaluates people and plans based on their personal characteristics rather than our own personal assumptions.[14,16,23]

Setting an agenda at the outset of a visit is a form of perspective-taking that helps clinicians avoid misunderstandings about expectations. It allows negotiation on how to optimally balance the priorities of both the patient and clinician. Eliciting the full list of patient concerns up front increases connection and self-efficacy for both patient and clinician.[15]

Open-ended questions can further elucidate perspective (eg, "How has this situation impacted you emotionally?" "What are your expectations about how I can help?"). It is useful to explore the person's ideas about what might be causing a given situation, the impact it has had on them, and expectations of what is hoped for as an outcome.

Improving Information-Sharing

Other core skills required for effective communication relate to providing information. Relationship-centered communication features the "Ask-Respond-Tell" (ART) model to identify patient's understanding of medical situations and options, attend to the emotional impact of such information, and actively engage patients in making a treatment plan.[17] ART provides information incrementally in small digestible portions; this improves efficiency by creating an engaging dialogue that can pivot and evolve to meet the needs of both parties rather than wasting time on information already known or with a "data download" of overwhelmingly large amounts of information. A specialized type of ART is often referred to as "teach-back" to check understanding (**Box 2**).[17] Teach-back maximizes the fidelity of information transfer, particularly with complex topics.

APPROACH TO LEARNING COMMUNICATION SKILLS
Independent Practice

An individual may study and review communication skills but that alone is insufficient for sustainable improvement. Context and authenticity are key for effective

---

Box 2
Example of a "teach-back" Ask-Respond-Tell loop

Clinician (Ask): I just went over a lot of information. To be sure we're on the same page, would you mind telling me your understanding of our plan from today?

Patient: OK. I need to check my blood sugar every morning, and if it's high, increase my insulin dose by 2 units. If it's good, then we'll keep the dose the same.

Clinician (Respond): Yes! That's correct! (Tell) We also talked about what to do if your sugar is too low. (Ask) What do you remember about that?

Patient: Well, I remember you said I should decrease my insulin dose, but I don't remember by how much.

Clinician (Respond): It's completely understandable—we talked about a lot of things. (Tell) We said that if your sugar was less than 80, you should decrease your insulin dose by 4 units. (Ask) What other questions do you have?

---

communication. Intentional practice is needed to gain both confidence in building microskills and understanding of patient responses to each strategy. When practicing individually, without the benefit of an experienced observer for feedback, it is helpful to have a *specific*, *achievable*, and *flexible* goal before entering a conversation. Invoking a goal targets the mind to a particular moment of a conversation, prompting preparation to learn a microskill (eg, ask for patient understanding before giving information) more deeply. The *specificity* encourages the development of thinking about communication as an objective skill that can be improved. An *achievable* goal should be reasonable within the context of the patient encounter; a 10-minute urgent care visit for sinusitis may *not* be the time to practice asking about end-of-life preferences. Finally, *flexibility* refers to the need to keep the patient at the focus of communication, adapting to their needs and feedback (perspective-taking). It is possible, for example, to reflect on an interaction with a patient in its immediate aftermath to assess how it went—what did I do effectively, and what would I want to modify the next time I interact with this patient or others?

Self-reflection is a powerful method to make incremental improvements in skills that are within one's own awareness. Although self-reflection often takes the form of ruminating about interactions after they have occurred, critical reflection more rigorously involves identifying and questioning assumptions about what happened in an interaction and applying lessons learned.[24] Audio/video recordings can augment this critical reflective practice and reduce recall bias.[25,26] However, improvement is limited by the individual's ability to recognize problems and potential for alternative outcomes without knowledge of advanced skill sets. These blind spots are, by definition, unseen, and illuminating them requires external feedback. In addition, communication is a social behavior; thus, methods to improve must incorporate socially based learning. Merely reading articles about communication is not enough to develop expertise. Deliberate practice and directed feedback from coaches, peers, or patients are needed to act as guides to foster self-regulation and problem-solving. Asking trusted external observers to host feedback conversations decreases blind spots and accelerates social learning of communication. For example, review of audio or video of a patient encounter (with the patient's explicit permission, of course) with a colleague, a communication coach (see section below), or patient advocate has the potential to augment learning through illumination of blind spots.

When reviewing patient encounters, clinicians can refer to cognitive frameworks that have been developed and well established by several groups and organizations

(**Table 3**). Connection with these or other professional organizations with courses for communication skill development is an additional way to obtain coaching and feedback. It also builds opportunities for mentorship and relationships with like-minded individuals to support skill development.

Individual Coaching

As noted previously, communication is a social activity, and thus independent practice only goes so far. Individual coaching and practice such as simulation or role play seem to produce the most effective learning and behavior change.[3] These teaching tools offer opportunities to practice in a psychologically safe learning environment, fostering skill development that may deepen one's learning more readily than in a real patient encounter where the stakes are higher for both clinician and patient. Individual and group coaching requires that all participants have a shared language and framework for communication skills in order to provide and receive meaningful feedback.[31]

Group Learning

Group learning further enhances the social aspect of improving communication skills. Several programs exist to develop expert facilitators for communication skill practice and feedback (see **Table 3**). The part of the patient can be played by another clinician,

Table 3	
Examples of communication cognitive frameworks	
Framework	**Sample Microskills**
Academy for Communication in Healthcare (ACH) Relationship Centered Communication (RCC)[27]	Create rapport quickly[15] Negotiate an agenda[15] Explore and respond to emotions with 'PEARLS' statements (P-Partnership; E-Naming Emotion; A-Appreciation; R-Respect; L-Legitimization; S-Support)[16] Share information in clear and concise way, assessing understanding with ART (A-Ask; R-Respond; T-Tell)[17] "Teach-back" for checking understanding[17]
'SPIKES' framework for breaking bad news[28]	S- Setting Up the Interview P- Assessing the Patients Perception I- Obtaining the patient's Invitation K- Giving Knowledge E- Addressing Emotion S- Strategy & Summary
Vital Talk organization's 'REMAP' framework for serious illness communication and 'NURSE' statements for expressing verbal empathy[29]	'REMAP' (R-Reframe; E-Emotion; M-Map Values; A-Align with values; P- Propose a Plan) 'NURSE' statements (N-Name; U-Understand; R-Respect; S-Support; E-Explore)
Ariadne Labs Serious Illness Conversation Guide[30]	Set up the conversation Assess understanding and preferences Share prognosis Explore key topics Close the conversation

a standardized or simulated patient, or possibly, under circumstances that do not interfere with their care, a real patient. For specific techniques and approaches to teaching communication skills, we refer the reader to additional resources and trainings.[32,33]

System-Based Approach

As an administrator or leader in health care, exemplary communication skills are essential. Many leaders may feel daunted by the prospect of how to change organizational culture to support a more person-centered atmosphere. Fortunately, use of communication microskills demonstrates effective leadership by example and creates an environment that respects and values its employees through fostering autonomy, collaboration, engagement, and open communication.[34] We list several examples of how to demonstrate effective leadership in communication in the following section.

To inspire culture change as a system, leaders must achieve staff buy-in toward any shared common goal. Although most health care workers would agree that communication skills with patients, families, and colleagues are an essential part of practice, merely mandating training constitutes an extrinsic motivator that may have limited effectiveness. In his transformational change model, Kotter invokes 2 areas where leadership can use foundational communication skills to affect change: elicit buy-in by perspective-taking of staff through close listening and understanding their pain points and develop a strategy to effectively communicate those perspectives with a growth mindset.[35]

Leaders can establish standards for communication in onboarding orientations and skills refreshers, in the form of ongoing coaching and/or repeat workshops, at regular intervals. There is a temptation to rely on online modules or "one-off" trainings; however, evidence shows that these methods do not lead to lasting effects.[36] Effective workshops must include skills practice, reinforcement, and direct feedback. Although resource intensive, investment can have significant benefits beyond patient satisfaction metrics. Providers who communicate in a relationship-centered manner have better clinical outcomes, which can translate into improved reimbursement, particularly in a value-based model.[7,37] Providers will also have greater job satisfaction, engagement, and improved retention.[34]

How an organization's leadership communicates sets the tone for its staff and workers. Therefore, leadership must "walk the talk" by engaging in the same workshops, level the hierarchy, and build a shared mental model around how all members of the organization communicate.[35] Leaders who are intentional in using the foundational microskills build trust with their employees through increased transparency, respect, and empathy.[38]

Although it is tempting to use clinical outcomes (eg, hemoglobin A1c, mortality rate) to assess the effect of communication improvement programs, many additional factors influence these "hard" clinical outcomes. Instead, educationally sensitive patient outcomes, which are intermediate or surrogate markers more strongly affected by education efforts, are useful.[39] For example, a patient's perception of their care experience has a positive correlation with clinical outcomes such as improved quality of life, self-efficacy, treatment adherence, and management of chronic diseases.[40–42] Consumer Assessment of Healthcare Providers & Systems (CAHPS) scores are used as a surrogate marker for the patient's perception. These scores can be influenced independently from a hospital or practice's performance by response bias, survey administration method, and case-mix.[43] Despite these limitations in using CAHPS scores as accurate measures of communication skill, they can be useful from an administrative or systems point of view for objective evaluation of practitioners and to target opportunities for improvement by providing patterns of patient experience to target specific problem areas that a provider or institution may need to address. In addition, value-based reimbursement is a powerful motivator for health systems to support communication skill–building initiatives.[7,37]

Another useful extrinsic metric is clinician satisfaction. Clinician burnout has become epidemic and creates barriers to effective patient care and work engagement. Evidence shows that clinicians who communicate using relationship-centered skills have an association with higher work satisfaction.[44] Discussion with providers on how their intrinsic motivators can be supported to create "ground-up" solutions, rather than "top-down," is more likely to succeed and be sustainable.

SUMMARY

Intrinsic and extrinsic motivators improve individual communication skills. Foundational skills improve with deliberate practice and feedback. Communication skills can improve on the individual, group, or systems level. Clinician communication skills excel through intentional reflection, an institutional focus on relationship-centered care, and ongoing skill development and support. Ultimately, the goal is not merely to make skills better (although naturally, that is desirable): it is also for development and enhancement of community, ongoing peer reinforcement of effective communication skills, and support of health care staff in the context of arduous work with high burnout risk. Through enhancing communication skills and thereby these individual and community connections, we can make the work of health care more sustainable, higher quality, and increasingly humanistic.

CLINICS CARE POINTS

---

1) After reflecting on interpersonal interactions, select a specific learning goal to improve communication skills. Consider a coach to observe in real time or to review an audio or video of an encounter.

2) Develop awareness of internal emotional reactions and implicit biases that ultimately affect patient outcomes.

3) For system-wide communication initiatives, select multiple methods of assessing success (eg, patient experience scores, narratives, 360-degree evaluations, clinician burnout) that encompass multiple perspectives.

DISCLOSURE

Dr C.L. Chou receives honoraria for teaching with the nonprofit academic organization Academy of Communication in Healthcare.

REFERENCES

1. Stewart MA. Effective physician-patient communication and health outcomes: a review. CMAJ 1995;152(9):1423–33.
2. Stewart M, Brown JB, Donner A, et al. The impact of patient-centered care on outcomes. J Fam Pract 2000;49(9):796–804.
3. Ericsson K, Prietula M, Cokely E. The making of an expert. Harv Bus Rev 2021. Available at: https://hbr.org/2007/07/the-making-of-an-expert. Accessed October 14 2021.
4. Ericsson K. Expertise. Curr Biol 2014;24(11):R508–10.

5. Deci EL, Ryan RM. Intrinsic motivation and self-determination in human behavior. 1st ed. Perspectives in social psychology, xvi. Boston, MA: Springer; 1985. p. 372.

6. Ryan RM, Deci EL. Self-determination theory and the facilitation of intrinsic motivation, social development, and well-being. Am Psychol 2000;55(1):68–78.

7. Boissy A, Windover AK, Bokar D, et al. Communication skills training for physicians improves patient satisfaction. J Gen Intern Med 2016;31(7):755–61.

8. Cook DA, Artino AR. Motivation to learn: an overview of contemporary theories. Med Educ 2016;50(10):997–1014.

9. Mueller CM, Dweck CS. Praise for intelligence can undermine children's motivation and performance. J Pers Soc Psychol 1998;75(1):33–52.

10. Deci EL, Koestner R, Ryan RM. A meta-analytic review of experiments examining the effects of extrinsic rewards on intrinsic motivation. Psychol Bull 1999;125(6): 627–68.

11. Deci EL. Effects of externally mediated rewards on intrinsic motivation. J Pers Soc Psychol 1971;18(1):05–115. https://doi.org/10.1037/h0030644.

12. Cameron J, Banko KM, Pierce WD. Pervasive negative effects of rewards on intrinsic motivation: the myth continues. Behav Analyst 2001;24(1):1–44.

13. Smith RC, Dwamena FC, Fortin AH. Teaching personal awareness. J Gen Intern Med 2005;20(2):201–7.

14. Devine PG, Forscher PS, Austin AJ, et al. Long-term reduction in implicit race bias: a prejudice habit-breaking intervention. J Exp Soc Psychol 2012;48(6): 1267–78.

15. Fortin AH, Mills L. Skill set one: the beginning of the encounter. In: Chou C, Cooley L, editors. Communication Rx. New York, NY: McGraw Hill; 2017.

16. Clark WD, Russell M. Skill set two: skills that build trust. In: Chou C, Cooley L, editors. Communication Rx. New York, NY: McGraw Hill; 2017.

17. Chou CM. Skill set three: delivering diagnoses and treatment plans. In: Chou C, Cooley L, editors. Communication Rx. New York, NY: McGraw Hill; 2017.

18. Greenwald AG, McGhee DE, Schwartz JL. Measuring individual differences in implicit cognition: the implicit association test. J Pers Soc Psychol 1998;74(6): 1464–80.

19. Rollnick S, Miller WR, Butler C. Motivational interviewing in health care: helping patients change behavior. Applications of motivational interviewing. New York, NY: Guilford Press; 2008. p. 210.

20. Rosenberg MB. A model for nonviolent communication. Third edition. Encinitas, CA: PuddleDancer Press; 2015. p. 264.

21. Kalet A, Chou CL. Remediation in medical education : a mid-course correction. New York, NY: Springer; 2014. p. 367.

22. Chou CL. Communication rx : transforming healthcare through relationship-centered communication. New York, NY: McGraw-Hill; 2018. p. 272.

23. Edgoose JYC, Quiogue M, Sidhar K. How to identify, understand, and unlearn implicit bias in patient care. Fam Pract Manag 2019;26(4):29–33.

24. Karnieli-Miller O. Reflective practice in the teaching of communication skills. Patient Educ Couns 2020;103(10):2166–72.

25. Hargie OD, Morrow NC. Using videotape in communication skills training: a critical evaluation of the process of self-viewing. Med Teach 1986;8(4):359–65.

26. Hammoud MM, Morgan HK, Edwards ME, et al. Is video review of patient encounters an effective tool for medical student learning? a review of the literature. Adv Med Educ Pract 2012;3:19–30.

27. Chou CL, Cooley L, Pearlman RE, et al. Enhancing patient experience by training local trainers in fundamental communication skills. Patient Experience J 2014; 1(2):8.

28. Baile WF, Buckman R, Lenzi R, et al. SPIKES—a six-step protocol for delivering bad news: application to the patient with cancer. Oncologist 2000;5(4):302–11.

29. Childers JW, Back AL, Tulsky JA, et al. REMAP: a framework for goals of care conversations. J Oncol Pract 2017;13(10):e844–50.

30. Lakin JR, Koritsanszky LA, Cunningham R, et al. A systematic intervention to improve serious illness communication in primary care. Health Aff 2017;36(7): 1258–64.

31. Ericsson KA. An expert-performance perspective of research on medical expertise: the study of clinical performance. Med Educ 2007;41(12):1124–30. https:// doi.org/10.1111/j.1365-2923.2007.02946.x.

32. Siropaides CH, Howell M, Chou CL. Teaching about emotions in healthcare. In: Schwartz R, Hall J, Osterberg L, editors. Emotion in the clinical encounter. New York, NY: McGraw Hill; 2021.

33. Pearlman RE. Teaching the skill sets. In: Chou C, Cooley L, editors. Communication Rx. New York, NY: McGraw Hill; 2017.

34. Tullar JM, Amick BC, Brewer S, et al. Improve employee engagement to retain your workforce. Health Care Manage Rev 2016;41(4):316–24.

35. Kotter JP. Leading change: why transformation efforts fail. Harv Bus Rev 2007;92–107.

36. Brown JB, Boles M, Mullooly JP, et al. Effect of clinician communication skills training on patient satisfaction. a randomized, controlled trial. Ann Intern Med 1999;131(11):822–9.

37. Yağar F. Why does patient–physician communication matter? more active patients, decreased healthcare use and costs. J Patient Experience 2021;8. 237437352110365.

38. Cunningham L. A tool kit for improving communication in your healthcare organization. Front Health Serv Manage Fall 2019;36(1):3–13.

39. Yin HS, Jay M, Maness L, et al. Health literacy: an educationally sensitive patient outcome. J Gen Intern Med 2015;30(9):1363–8.

40. Sequist TD, Schneider EC, Anastario M, et al. Quality monitoring of physicians: linking patients' experiences of care to clinical quality and outcomes. J Gen Intern Med 2008;23(11):1784–90.

41. Wanzer MB, Booth-Butterfield M, Gruber K. Perceptions of health care providers' communication: relationships between patient-centered communication and satisfaction. Health Commun 2004;16(3):363–83.

42. Heisler M, Bouknight RR, Hayward RA, et al. The relative importance of physician communication, participatory decision making, and patient understanding in diabetes self-management. J Gen Intern Med 2002;17(4):243–52.

43. Elliott MN, Zaslavsky AM, Goldstein E, et al. Effects of survey mode, patient mix, and nonresponse on CAHPS hospital survey scores. Health Serv Res 2009;44(2 Pt 1):501–18.

44. Krasner MS, Epstein RM, Beckman H, et al. Association of an educational program in mindful communication with burnout, empathy, and attitudes among primary care physicians. JAMA 2009;302(12):1284–93.

Printed and bound by CPI Group (UK) Ltd, Croydon, CR0 4YY

03/10/2024

01040476-0014